The University of Wisconsin Medical School
A Chronicle, 1848–1948

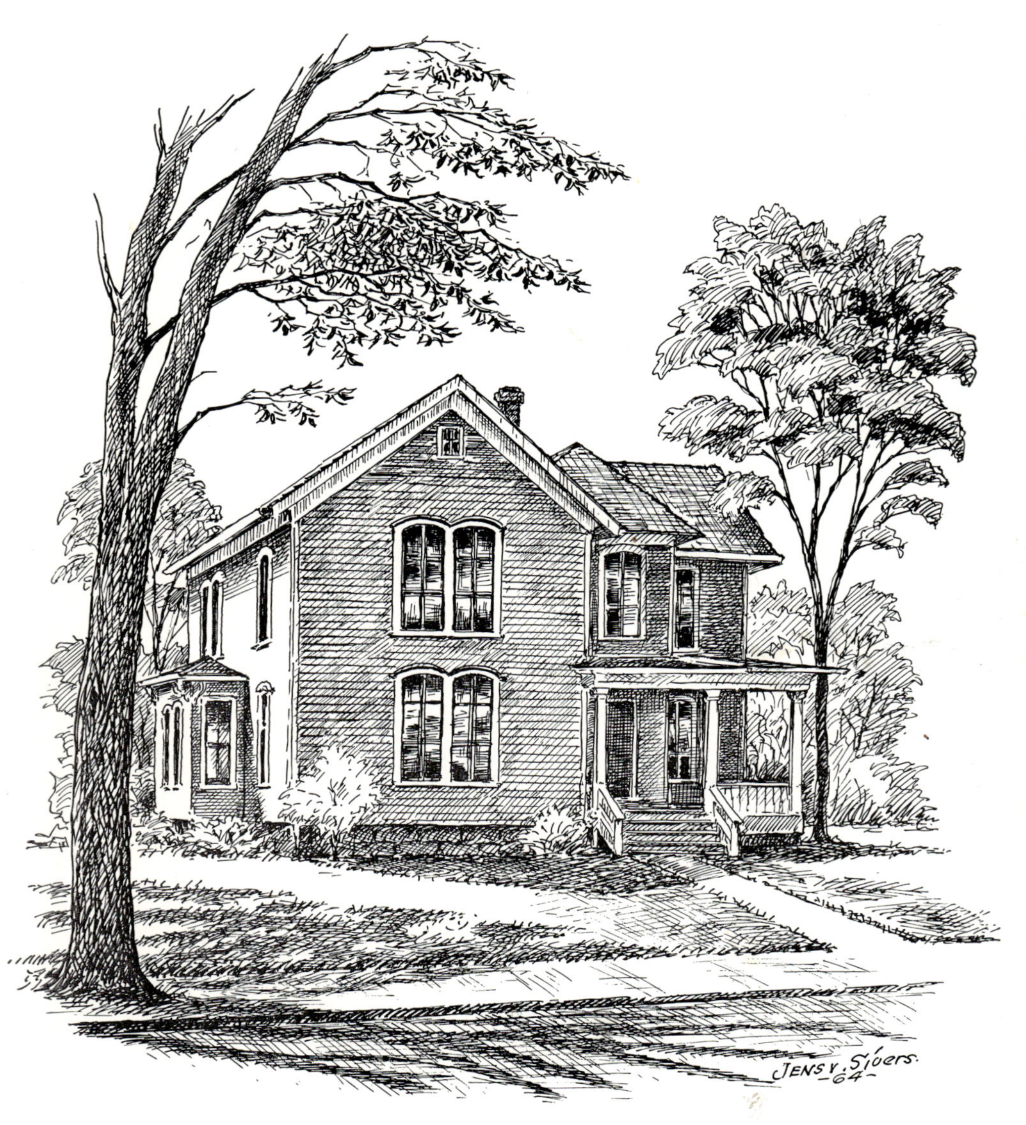

Cornelius House, first student clinic

The University of Wisconsin Medical School

A Chronicle, 1848-1948

Paul F. Clark

Emeritus Professor of Medical Microbiology

*Published for the Wisconsin Medical
Alumni Association by
The University of Wisconsin Press*

MADISON, MILWAUKEE, AND LONDON, 1967

Published for
The Wisconsin Medical Alumni Association
by the University of Wisconsin Press
Madison, Milwaukee, and London
U.S.A.: Box 1379, Madison, Wisconsin 53701
U.K.: 26–28 Hallam Street, London, W.1

Printed in the United States of America by
North Central Publishing Company
St. Paul, Minnesota

Library of Congress Catalog Card Number 67–12004

Foreword

The Medical School is a comparatively youthful member of the academic family. Although the act of incorporation of the University, signed by Governor Nelson Dewey, July 26, 1848, listed medicine among its four authorized departments, nearly sixty years elapsed before its inception. The long delay in fulfilling the mandate of the legislature while all neighboring states met this educational need in itself would invite careful study. However, in a constructive sense, attention to the undaunted courage of men of vision should prevail over the temptation to explore the trials and frustrations of the protracted gestational period of the Medical School.

After the abortive gesture of the "paper faculty" of the 1850's, the first movement toward the initiation of a medical curriculum on the University campus was the Special Course Antecedent to Medicine (1887). The quality of this course and its successor, the Premedical Course (1890), laid a firm foundation for the establishment, first, of the preclinical two-year course (1907) and, then, the complete four-year course (1925). Before the evolution of clinical facilities in the University, Wisconsin men and women completing their undergraduate medical education and hospital training in the great medical centers of the country frequently remained in these areas. Many of these transplanted Badgers attained scientific and professional eminence in their respective fields. In effect, these "intellectual hostages" vastly strengthened their adopted medical communities; but, by the same token, they abstracted their potential contributions from their native state.

Regardless of this circumstance, the native sons and daughters of Wisconsin are conspicuously loyal. When the Wisconsin Medical Alumni Association took its present organized form, it immediately sought channels to express its deep interest in the Medical School. Among the first deficiencies encountered was the lack of a history of their Alma Mater. With the passage of time the faces and forms of their teachers were becoming less distinct. The ringing voices of the classroom and the laboratory were less clear. Could the rapport with the faculty have been as intimate as they recalled, or was it a vagary of memory? The old familiar haunts had disappeared. And were the laboratories in the attics and basements of Science Hall and the old Chemical Engineering Building quite as makeshift as they seemed in an earlier day? Appreciating the magnitude of the task and at the same time realizing that time would increase rather than diminish its arduousness, the Committee recommended that the Association undertake the preparation of the history of the Medical School. The Association enthusiastically voted to supply clerical and stenographic support for this project.

The selection of Professor Emeritus Paul F. (for Fish Kettle to generations of disrespectful medical students!) Clark as historian was a particularly happy one. Highly regarded as a teacher and scientist, he holds an impeccable position in the academic world. A strict disciplinarian in the classroom and laboratory, he is a man of easy friendship and warmth of personality which open many avenues of communication. Arriving on the Wisconsin scene in 1914, he lived through the lean years that tried the mettle of men. Yet he would be the first to grant that it is an unusual privilege to attend and participate in the birth and rearing of a medical school. No faculty member can be more proud of the Wisconsin product. Were the Committee to have scrutinized Dr. Clark's literary qualifications, several attributes would have arrested their attention. Certainly his whimsical turn in *Alice in Virusland* (1938) would have attracted their notice. Meticulous care in detail marked *Memorable Days in Medicine: A Calendar of Biology and Medicine* (1942), written with Mrs. Clark. His *Pioneer Microbiologists of America* (1961) is a classic account of the lives and contributions of our scientists in this field. By personal touches and literary allusions, and with fine artistry, Dr. Clark has made his subjects live and breathe on the written page.

Having assumed this assignment, for over two years Dr. Clark has lent his fine talents and great energy to the task of collecting data from innumerable sources. Letters from alumni and friends of the Medical School have greatly enriched his pool of information. "Like the parson's attic, he refuses nothing." Such material was then welded into workable form for ultimate refinement and organization for writing. With the privilege of a preview of the manuscript, I would describe it as a remarkably faithful account of the development of our Medical School. Such problems as arose are dealt with dispassionately and without acerbity or rancor. The vignettes of his fellow faculty members are drawn with a facile pen. Almost they speak for themselves. If there were a single minuscule of reservation in his characterizations, it may be paraphrased from Matthew Prior:

> Be to [their] virtues very kind;
> Be to [their] faults a little blind.

Dr. Clark has wrought a splendid lasting documentary account of the University of Wisconsin Medical School. Assuredly, it will take its proper place in the archives of our great Medical School and University as a milestone of reference. Laboring without remuneration, the author demonstrates his dedication and sense of responsibility in this major *Arbeit*. Only a New Englander — "Mainiac," he terms himself — could have achieved his objective. Generations of Wisconsin men and women will be grateful to the Wisconsin Medical Alumni Association for its promulgation and support of this project and to Dr. Clark for his prodigious efforts in its surpassing execution.

Madison, Wisconsin   WILLIAM S. MIDDLETON
March, 1966

Preface

To the directors and members of the University of Wisconsin Medical Alumni Association, we all owe gratitude for this history. To Mischa Lustok and Einar Daniels, who were the ones who dreamed up this affair and gave it the initial push, all who may cherish this history are greatly indebted.

For about three years, I have been striving to follow the wishes of the alumni as expressed in a letter of January 6, 1964, from Dr. Mischa Lustok, then president of the University of Wisconsin Medical Alumni Association. They urged me to write the "history of the Medical School from the vantage point of personal experience and human relationships," a family history rather than one of statistics.

Their letter necessarily set the broad standards; I have had to establish certain others. I have used the Regents' seven-year period for "tenure" as my criterion for the minimum number of years of faculty service necessary for inclusion in the history. Commonly, I have omitted consideration of the families of the faculty, a practice usual in histories of medical schools and universities. Lists of honors so readily available in scientific and public directories have been excluded. They make for dreary reading and I am not competing with *Who's Who*.

Names of the residents in the several departments of the hospital are given in the appropriate chapters about the Medical School. This type of instruction and practice has high importance in affecting the quality of medical practice throughout the state and the country, and our residents bear the stamp of this Medical School even though they have earned their medical degrees from other institutions. Records are incomplete but, despite errors, I have tried to give the terminal date of the service of each man as a resident.

The term "department" has been used loosely by almost everyone in the Medical School, referring to a recognized discipline rather than to a "department" legally created by action of the University Board of Regents. I have commonly followed custom rather than legal detail. Through the decades the different disciplines have usually worked well together whatever the organization has been. The major difference is that the chairman of a department becomes a member of the Executive Committee of the school and may take a stronger part in policy decisions.

The directors of the alumni association who initiated this project and their successors have cheerfully supported the task in providing funds to employ student secretarial aid and search in the University Archives. I owe so much to so many others who have given aid that only those who have helped exceptionally can be mentioned here. Many who have written letters and those with whom I have held conferences are cited with appreciation in the notes. I have deeply appreciated the many warm letters from former students and faculty who have shown such encouraging interest in this history. These letters and other materials collected for this history will be placed in the University Archives.

I am deeply grateful to Frances E. Holford, Nikolaus Mani, William S. Middleton, and Charles V. Seastone, who have read the entire manuscript, given helpful criticisms, and pulled me out of the undertow of the full moon tides. For repeated help, I am indebted to Harold C. Bradley, Garrett A. Cooper, Helen Crawford, Helen A. Dickie, Joseph W. Gale, Ralph A. Hawley, Harry M. Kay, Chauncey D. Leake, Ovid O. Meyer, Otto A. Mortensen, Harland W. Mossman, William H. Oatway, Jr., Karver L. Puestow, Jackman Pyre, Hans H. Reese, Robert J. Samp, H. Kent Tenney, Jr., Ralph M. Waters, Herman W. Wirka, and William B. Youmans. Mrs. Walter Schulte (Helen Denne), Helen L. Bunge, and Marjorie C. Paquin gave aid in writing the chapter on the University of Wisconsin School of Nursing and Nursing Services. Several members of Dr. Bardeen's family have been generously helpful. Most of the photographs have come from Homer Montague and the staff of the University Medical Center photographic laboratory. Student secretarial aides have come and gone; I can mention only the one who served longest, Patricia Progre, and also Sylvia Wallace, who did much searching in the University Archives.

Bibliographic materials have been cited in the notes. Mr. J. E. Boell, University Archivist, and his well-indexed archives of letters, Regents' records, and reports of presidents and deans have been invaluable. The University catalogues have constituted a printed record of great importance. Because the last catalogue in our period covered 1948–50, I have commonly included those two extra years in the history. Alden White, University Secretary of Faculty, and Mrs. Betty Smith of his staff have provided me promptly with the detailed records of the life histories and University appointments of the faculty.

The historians of our University, Merle Curti and Vernon Carstensen, have been my mentors not only through their critical sympathetic published history of the University (1848–1925), but also through personal advice. Each of them has agreed that since I have been on the faculty for more than half a century, I have become a "primary source" and may use the first person singular as I see fit. The department of medical microbiology has provided space for this work as well as many other welcome aids.

To Alice Schiedt Clark, my helpmate for well beyond the golden wedding period, I owe, as always, appreciation beyond my capacity to express; she has given needed encouragement and daily editorial readings and corrections throughout the whole course of this work.

For me this has been a labor of love and, as such, it has been a mixture of pain and pleasure. Collecting the material, thinking of you all, and remembering my early colleagues, warm friends, most of them gone, has been a great joy and a rare privilege for one in his middle eighties. The many decisions essential in the writing have at times been painful.

After reading scores of accounts of conflicts, both within and without the University, and considering these in the light of my own experience, I have concluded that it is really remarkable that our Medical School was ever born and even more remarkable that it has continued to grow through two terrible world wars and a disastrous period of depression to a medical center of distinction. The whole history has been one of democracy in action and, as such, is a most encouraging story.

Were there "giants in those days" or is that notion the happy perspective of years? Yes, I think there were one or two "giants in those days," such as Charles Russell Bardeen and Joseph Spragg Evans. There were also a number of other men of splendid character, enthusiasms, and achievement. I hope you will enjoy the necessarily too brief and possibly not too highly objective vignettes of these men that I have, with the help of others, been able to paint. I beg your forgiveness for my errors of omission and commission.

"I am a part of all that I have met"; I am, therefore, a part of you and you are a part of me.

Ave atque vale

Madison, Wisconsin   PAUL F. CLARK
October, 1966

Contents

CONTENTS

Illustrations

The University of Wisconsin Medical School
A Chronicle, 1848–1948

1 Acceptance of the Challenge

Come, we will transform the world by our discoveries.
Pasteur

Early in March, 1904, the North Western Railroad noon train from Chicago rumbled into the busy Madison station, at the corner of Blair and King streets, and screeched to a stop. Several dozen persons hurried off the train; among them was a somewhat rumpled, square-built man of average height, about thirty years of age, who climbed down from the smoking car with his pipe well clutched in his teeth. He looked about him, obviously expecting to be met, and from the considerable group of waiting spectators appeared a small dignified man, apparently in his forties, dressed with meticulous neatness. After warm greetings, the two men — the younger still carrying his bag — walked slowly out to King Street and caught a waiting trolley car. Of course, at this date, there were no automobiles, but one or two hacks and a number of horse-drawn trucks were busy around the station. Up King Street and around the Capitol the trolley car clanged its way, its interior slightly warmer than the outside air, because of a small, glowing coal stove in the corner. A five-cent fare took our new acquaintances to the University, where they got off and climbed up Bascom Hill, still slippery from the winter snows. The two men had much in common and much to talk about. They were both anatomists and both had been students of Franklin Mall, the outstanding professor of anatomy at Johns Hopkins Medical School. Both men knew that their meeting that day might be the first step toward the founding of a new medical school at the University of Wisconsin. In Bascom Hall they made their way to President Van Hise's office and there our visitor was warmly greeted and remained closeted with the president for a considerable period.

Just a year before this meeting, the Regents of the University, after considerable hesitation, had elected the forceful Charles R. Van Hise, prominent member of the geology department, to the presidency. The founding of a medical school, so long a tenuous dream, was one of Van Hise's major objectives. He pushed it, as he did all his projects, with characteristic drive. In December of 1903 he had made a trip to Philadelphia and Baltimore to find a man to become professor of anatomy and a leader in establishing a new medical school. Among several excellent men, he was especially taken with Dr. Mall's protégé, Charles R. Bardeen, an associate professor of anatomy at Johns Hopkins who had been making quite a name for himself in embryology. It was this young man who was greeted on that March day in 1904 by Dr. William Snow Miller, then an assistant professor in the biology department.

Unfortunately, we have no record of the conversation between Van Hise and Bardeen, only the official record of his appointment as professor of anatomy in 1904. We do, however, have three warmly appreciative letters from Bardeen to Miller written in March and April, 1904. In Bardeen's letter to Miller on March 18, 1904, he states, "I have accepted the position offered me at Madison and together, I feel sure we can build up a strong department of anatomy. . . . Later in the spring I expect to pay another visit at Madison, and we can then talk things over and plan an aggressive campaign for the development of the department." In his letter of March 24, 1904, he says, "I can assure you that I have only admiration and wonder for all you have done under the hampered conditions in which you have worked." He says much about plans for anatomy, but not a word about the possibility of a medical school.

During the next two years, however, both Bardeen and Van Hise were extraordinarily active. In 1905–6, Van Hise presented for Regent approval Bardeen's outline of a two-year medical course that could be offered by the University. When the legislature met in 1907, the president requested not only additional funds for the University but also approval of the two-year medical school. Despite opposition from many sides, the appropriation bill containing this authorization was passed by both houses with substantial majorities. At long last we were on the road, though it proved a long and winding route.

Let's take a look for a moment at Madison and the University during those early years of the 1900's when Bardeen and Van Hise were inviting promising young men to join in the founding of a new medical school. Manifestly this is not a history, merely a few glimpses into that period so vastly different from today. The differences are so great that we can hardly appreciate the early problems of the Medical School without picturing something of that era.

Van Hise had come into the presidency on the crest of a wave. The half-century jubilee, which had been planned for several years, was celebrated in 1904 with enthusiasm. Delegates from major universities and learned societies in both Europe and the United States came to express their interest in and respect for our growing university. Many speeches were read and some thirty-nine honorary degrees were conferred.

The one degree of special interest to us, and the only one to a medical man, was that awarded to Franklin P. Mall of Johns Hopkins University.

FRANKLIN PAINE MALL: Foremost investigator in anatomy in America, leader in recent advance in medical education, you have established productive departments of anatomy in three universities. Your teaching has inspired a strong group of disciples doing important investigative work at this and other universities. You are well worth the honor of all, for your aim is to decrease human suffering. This university therefore confers upon you the degree of Doctor of Laws.[1]

We are particularly interested in Mall because he was the stimulating teacher not only of William Snow Miller, back at Clark University, but also of Charles R. Bardeen, who was to become the first dean and wise leader of the Medical School.

The Madison of those Jubilee days seems far removed from the city we see today. In praise, our University poet, William Ellery Leonard, wrote:

> 'Tis no mean city: When I shut my eyes,
> To thought, she seems memorial as they,
> The world's white cities famous far away,
> With her own beauty, her own sunset skys
> Across her waters, her own enterprise
> Beside her woodlands, with her thousand homes,
> Her squares and flowering parks, and those two domes
> Of Law and Learning, and her bold and wise.[2]

But not all was so poetically idyllic. Indeed, in order to meet the demands of "Law and Learning," Madison quickly became a bustling, turn-of-the-century town. It was an important railway center, with three major companies — the Chicago and North Western Railroad, the Chicago, Milwaukee, and St. Paul Railroad, and the Illinois Central Railroad — providing public transportation in all directions.

In 1900 Madison boasted five banks, three daily newspapers, twenty-one churches, and seventy-two incorporated companies. Seven years later there were thirty churches and nearly one hundred and fifty incorporated companies. The population had grown from 19,500 to over 25,000. The busy city market place was at the beginning of East Washington Avenue, underneath a rather beautiful old water tower which was no longer in use. Farmers brought their produce, hay, and wood to sell, and buyers from Chicago and Milwaukee came to dicker for horses with local farmers at the monthly horse sales.

To many a new student entering the University, Madison seemed a big city. The boys found lodging in any of several rooming houses in the city or in fraternities and private homes. The standard charge for board was three dollars a week. Chadbourne, or Ladies' Hall, the only University dormitory, housed many of the coeds.

At the time of the beginning of the Medical School in 1907, Breese Terrace was a rural boundary and University Heights was just beginning to attract faculty householders. Lawyer Buell's house was the first, in 1894, Professor Ely's the second, in 1895, and Professor Knowlton's the third. Nakoma and Shorewood were farmland, and Maple Bluff a handful of summer cottages.

Looking at the larger scene, this was a period of exuberant optimism for the nation. The Spanish-American War and the capture of the Philippines had forced us to become a world power, although many Americans regarded the new responsibilities with mixed feelings. Industry was forging ahead and new opportunities were abundant. America's world-wide connections brought new markets abroad for American products, and the prosperity that had begun in the late 1890's, after a severe depression earlier in the decade, continued. Growth stimulated more growth. The farmers shared in the general prosperity; higher prices for their products encouraged many to purchase more land and new machinery.

Despite the farmers' prosperity, the dominant trend of the era was toward urbanization. In 1860, only 17 per cent of the American population lived in cities; by 1900, some 40 per cent of the 76,000,000 Americans were city dwellers. The growth of cities continued at an ever-accelerating pace, and the center of American population moved westward from the Atlantic coast.

Contributing to the general population growth and to urbanization were large waves of immigrants. America beckoned as a land of oppor-

tunity, and the peak of immigration came in the twentieth century before World War I. By 1910, one-third of the American people were
foreign-born or had parents born abroad. Most of the immigrants found
jobs in the cities or in the mining or railroad industries. The poorest and
lowest-paid jobs fell to the immigrants, and few workers of the 1900's
were highly paid. In 1900, factory, railroad, and mining employees received less than thirteen dollars for a fifty-nine-hour week. It is obvious
that not all shared in the prosperity of the era.

Americans felt that more should share in this prosperity. They recognized flaws in their society and felt that recognition of evil was the first
step toward reform. Child labor was a shocking problem in the early part
of the century; Professor E. A. Ross of the sociology department used to
declaim:

> The golf links lie so near the mill
> That almost every day
> The laboring children can look out
> And see the men at play.[3]

Muckrakers publicized the dangers of big business and corruption in city,
state, and national government. Reforming politicians at all levels experimented with new forms of government. Cities tried city managers; states
introduced the referendum, initiative, recall, and direct primary. State
and national leaders instituted more effective regulation of railroads, of
other business corporations, and of the food and drug industries.

Recognition of the value of scientific research increased, especially
in the universities and the new industrial laboratories. Educational facilities expanded, and changes in curriculum brought new, higher
standards. The circulation of newspapers and magazines grew rapidly.
People flocked to hear the Chautauqua lecturers and read Mr. Dooley's
(Finley Peter Dunne) penetrating and humorous Irish comments on the
contemporary scene. More and more Americans sent their children to
college.

The University and state of Wisconsin led in many of the new directions. Under Governor Robert M. La Follette, elected in 1900, Wisconsin enacted progressive legislation increasing state control over railroads,
lumbering, and other industries. La Follette was an intimate friend and
classmate of Van Hise, a fact that helped make real the latter's slogan,
"The boundaries of the University campus are the boundaries of the
state." At the University, leaders developed the "Wisconsin Idea" of

close cooperation between University and state groups and began using faculty experts in government, the farm, industry, and the home.[4] Under the leadership of Van Hise, the University continued to expand. In 1901, 2777 students attended, while the University had a total faculty of 180. By 1910, 4947 students worked under a faculty of 454. Thus, our Medical School was born in an era of dynamic growth and change for the University and the nation.

2   Early Steps

O brave new world, that has such people in't!
THE TEMPEST

We shall now drop back another half-century to examine briefly the first concept of the University of Wisconsin and a Medical School as one of its divisions. The territory of Wisconsin was hewn from the great Northwest Territory in 1836, and the first session of the territorial legislature passed an act authorizing the creation of a university to be supported by the territory. Although a board of trustees was named, no more came of the plan. In 1838, the legislature created a university of the territory of Wisconsin and provided it with two townships of land. We find the following pertinent sections of the act passed in 1838.

Section 1. Be it enacted by the council and house of representatives of the territory of Wisconsin, that there shall be established at or near Madison, the seat of government, a university for the purpose of educating youth, the name whereof shall be "the University of Wisconsin." The said university shall be under the government of a board of visitors not exceeding twenty-one in number.

Section 5. The said visitors may from time to time establish such colleges, academies and schools, depending upon the said university, as they may think proper and as the funds of the corporation will permit.

This act and land grant were the seeds from which the university idea grew.

Ten years later, on May 29, 1848, Wisconsin was admitted as the thirtieth state in the Union. The state constitution provided for the establishment of a university, and on July 26, 1848, Governor Nelson Dewey approved the act incorporating the University of Wisconsin. Two sections of that act are highly important.

9

Section 1. There shall be established in the state at or near the village of Madison in the county of Dane an institution of higher learning under the name and style of the University of Wisconsin.

Section 8. The University shall consist of four departments; First, the department of science, literature and the arts; second, the department of law; third, the department of medicine; fourth, the department of the theory and practice of elementary instruction.

The land grants made by the federal government for university purposes were vital in keeping such ideas alive. In those early days, general interest in the university idea was faint; it is obvious that in frontier communities, local schools were more immediately important. Despite many dissensions, a preparatory department was opened in the fall of 1848. In 1850, John Lathrop, the first chancellor of the University, was inaugurated, and North Hall, the first building, was erected.

University historians emphasize that from the time of the first land grant of the federal government sixty or more years elapsed before the University of Wisconsin could even begin to merit that name. There was little agreement in the early days about what a state university should be or do. The small faculty, meager funds, and clashing interests gave feeble support; the calamity of the Civil War drained away many students. For years, the larger part of the enrollment was in the preparatory department. After serious discord, this department was abolished during President Bascom's administration in 1880. Obviously, with the continuation and support of the University sometimes in jeopardy, the dream of adding a medical school had little immediate chance.

A welcome possibility arose on June 1, 1886, when a committee of five members of the State Medical Society headed by Dr. John M. Dodson of Delafield requested a meeting with the Regents of the University "in regard to establishing a preliminary course of medical study (it being understood that this is not to be a Medical Department in any sense of the word)." [1] The Regents responded favorably, and the new president, Thomas C. Chamberlin, who had the vision of a great university, also gave his approval. In the catalogue of 1887 appeared the announcement:

SPECIAL SCIENCE COURSE, ANTECEDENT TO THE STUDY OF MEDICINE

In response to a request from the Wisconsin State Medical Society, the University offers the following Special Course in Science, arranged for those contemplating the study of medicine and surgery. It is intended to give a broad and solid foundation for the professional course, together with collegiate culture.

The Chicago College of Physicians and Surgeons, Rush Medical College, and the Chicago Medical College have approved the course and will accept it as the equivalent of one year's study, thus enabling those who have taken the four years' course here to complete their medical course in these excellent colleges in two years.

All the studies given cannot be taken in the time allotted. Three full studies are required during each term, which may be chosen from those given. If the degree of Bachelor of Science is sought, the required studies of the General Science Course must be taken.

From the branches offered, special students may select a two years' course embracing the larger portion of those subjects which bear directly upon the studies of medicine and surgery. A more liberal course, however, is recommended, which shall embrace not only all of these sciences, but cognate branches and a due measure of language and of mental science, substantially as outlined in the following course.

The required subjects included zoology, vertebrate anatomy, histology, physiology, and bacteriology; until 1890, all of these courses, a tremendous load, were given by Professor Edward Birge. In 1888, twenty-seven students were registered in the premedical course and in 1892 this more specific name was adopted. The vital part that Birge, and after 1902, William Snow Miller played in these early steps towards a complete medical course should be heralded with appreciation. With little equipment and meager financial support, they instilled high ideals of excellence and accuracy. The students — such as Joseph C. Bloodgood and Albert J. Ochsner — were so well trained in histology and embryology that they were used as teachers in these subjects in the medical schools in which they were enrolled as students.

The teaching of bacteriology at the University had begun in 1884, three years before the start of the premedical program, in the botany department under William Trelease. The excitement of bacteriology had burst on all our colleges and universities about the same time, although a little earlier along the Atlantic seaboard. In institutions where there was no medical school, bacteriology was commonly first taught as a small offering in an already recognized field, such as botany or zoology.

By dint of proddings on the part of Trelease, some four hundred dollars' worth of apparatus to advance the work in bacteriology had been ordered, but did not arrive until after his departure to the Shaw Botanical Gardens of St. Louis. It fell, therefore, to Edward A. Birge, by this time professor of zoology, to unpack the treasure. As Birge told the medical students in 1935 in a talk on the beginnings of the premedical course in Wisconsin, "It was quite unthinkable that an equipment so large and valuable should stand idle, and so I was told to get busy and teach bacteriology, which accordingly I proceeded to do. I regarded my part in it as a temporary affair, so the course was not listed for the first two years. But Professor Charles R. Barnes, who succeeded Trelease in 1887, knew little and cared less about bacteria, so I, who meanwhile had learned a little about them, was obliged to continue the course."

The first specific appointment in bacteriology came in 1893; Harry Luman Russell became an assistant professor in bacteriology in the College of Agriculture with duties also in the Experiment Station. Through his responsibilities for all dairy products in the Agricultural Experiment Station, Russell became vitally interested in cattle. In 1894, Russell published the results of his application of the tuberculin test to cattle. He had injected a number of the cows of the Station with tuberculin primarily as a demonstration of the value of this test for his course students. At the beginning of the test there was no clinical evidence of tuberculosis in the herd, although during the test period one cow did show swelling of the udder and later physical signs of tuberculosis. Nevertheless, twenty-five of the thirty cattle reacted positively, twenty-two to the first test and three others to a later test. William A. Henry, dean of the College of Agriculture, and Russell decided not to temporize. All of the herd save two nonreactors were slaughtered and autopsied. The postmortem studies showed that every reacting cow and also one nonreacting animal had tuberculous lesions. This demonstration and similar tests carried out on other herds had tremendous influence throughout the state. Of course, there was violent conflict as to the accuracy of the test. In this case, also, the financial losses to the farmer were enormous in heavily infected herds. This whole story is a dramatic one and involved the forces in public health throughout the country. The control of bovine tuberculosis in the United States was an outstanding achievement in medical history.

Although the story of the several unsuccessful efforts to establish medical schools in different areas of Wisconsin has slight relation to the actual beginning of our school, we are happy to pay tribute to a number of men who were so persistent. Of these, we might mention Chandler B. Chapman, who tried to found a school in Madison and also in Rock Island, Illinois, and Alfred L. Castleman, who in the 1850's was dean of a medical department in the University of Wisconsin that never existed save on paper. The efforts made to establish medical schools have been well described in papers by William Snow Miller and by William S. Middleton.[2]

In the country at large, medical education and medical practice were in the doldrums throughout the early centuries with only an occasional school of distinction and only a few physicians who studied with adequately trained masters either in this country or in Europe. In his vividly told history of medicine in the United States, Morris Fishbein states:

> In a pioneer country, with a rapidly increasing population and the continued westward migration, the demand for doctors, and therefore for medical schools, was great. There were virtually no legal restrictions on the establishment of medical schools. Many were decidedly inferior and were established primarily for the financial gain of the promoters and the faculty. The operation of a medical school was often a profitable enterprise and there was an intense competition for students. Besides the so-called medical schools and the apprentice training in physicians' offices, there arose "diploma mills" in all sections of the country. These sold diplomas with no pretense whatsoever of providing medical training of any kind.
> The multiplication of medical schools was such that, by the end of the nineteenth century there were about as many medical schools in the United States as there were in all the rest of the world. A few of these institutions were of good quality . . . but chaos was the rule. . . . Admission requirements were usually nonexistent. Often ability to read and write was not essential.[3]

Henry Sigerist, professor of the history of medicine at Johns Hopkins, writes that "wherever a few doctors were gathered together, they could found a school, get a charter, call themselves professors, give medical instruction in some rented building, deal out diplomas, and pocket the tuition fees."[4]

Here in Wisconsin a single sentence from Middleton's paper tells the same story: "Irregular practice was rampant in the new state and, when every manner of practitioner was accepted at face value without reference to his qualifications and motivations, it required high courage to lead the fight against the forces of evil."[5] We must keep in mind that the state had no licensing board for physicians until 1897.

The basic need for well-trained physicians, the success of the premedical course, and the changes the new discoveries in bacteriology were causing in medicine and daily life were all factors in promoting the idea of developing a medical school within the University. However, it took the drive and skill of Van Hise and Bardeen to win over the Regents and the legislature and make the dream a reality.

3   The Beginning of the Attic Medical School

With all deductions, the triumphs of sanitary reform as well as of medical science are perhaps the brightest page in the history of our century.

W. E. H. Lecky

With Bardeen's appointment as professor of anatomy in 1904, it became obvious that at least a two-year medical school was being contemplated, although that was not publicly admitted. The momentous decision was made by the Regents and by the legislature in 1907. A bill establishing a College of Medicine weathered stormy debate and was passed by substantial majorities in both houses; it was signed by Governor Davidson on June 27, 1907. Initially, grounds for opposition centered around the idea that adequate medical instruction could be given only in large centers of population such as Milwaukee. Dr. William H. Washburn, dean of the Wisconsin College of Physicians and Surgeons in Milwaukee, quite naturally emphasized this idea and opposed the establishment of another medical school in Wisconsin, urging that there were already too many medical schools in our country, many of them inferior.[1] Washburn had ample evidence both from American Medical Association committees and from private agencies to support his contention that there were at that time an excessive number of inadequate proprietary medical schools in our country. Washburn hoped that the University would take over his school. Instead, in 1913, the Wisconsin College of Physicians and Surgeons joined Marquette Medical School, which later became a top-ranking institution.

The idea that the University would foster an inferior medical school was soon dispelled. The emphatic statements by Van Hise and by Bardeen that the University would never think of developing the clinical years without adequate hospital facilities under its own control silenced much of that opposition. The great value of developing a medical school in university surroundings with close relations to the underlying sciences, as well as the humanities, was emphasized by men important in medical education such as Dr. William H. Welch, dean of Johns Hopkins Medical School, and by Dr. Arthur D. Bevan, chairman of the American Medical Association Council on Medical Education. Since this council for years had been studying and encouraging improved medical education in our country, a statement from its chairman exerted great influence. He wrote:

I have had the opportunity this year of studying rather closely the conditions of medical education in this country. We have made a study of the conditions of medical education in each state. We have been much interested in studying the situation in Wisconsin and in the effort which the University of Wisconsin is making to establish a high grade medical course, or rather the first two years of the medical course.

We have found, that the great needs of medical education in this country are proper laboratory facilities and proper laboratory training in the sciences, which are taught in the first two years of a four year medical course. The establishment of a high grade course, such as the University of Wisconsin contemplates and would evidently develop would do very much to elevate the standards of medical education in your state.

The inspection of the medical colleges of the country, which was made this year by our committee, convinced all of us of the necessity of state control and state aid for modern medical education. A state cannot secure a high standard of medical practitioners without such aid and control. I believe that Wisconsin could not spend money which would bring her in greater returns than money intelligently spent in securing a high grade of medical practitioners, educated in her own state university.[2]

Letters from the Board of Medical Examiners both in Wisconsin and in neighboring states and from a long list of Milwaukee physicians favorably disposed to the idea of a university medical school greatly helped the situation. Dr. A. J. Patek, editor of the *Wisconsin Medical Journal*, and the prominent surgeon Dr. Albert J. Ochsner of Chicago also gave valuable aid. After Van Hise showed that our neighboring states all had publicly financed medical schools, the feeling that Wisconsin ought also to provide its young citizens with medical education finally prevailed.

This authorization of the two-year school gave Dean Bardeen and President Van Hise the challenging opportunity of choosing a faculty for the new school. With the approval of Van Hise and the Regents, Joseph Erlanger had been appointed professor of physiology and physiological chemistry in 1906, a year before the legislative approval of the two-year school. Erlanger, formerly associate professor of physiology at the Johns Hopkins Medical School, proved to be a remarkable choice. To our regret, he remained at Wisconsin only four years, after which he went to Washington University in St. Louis, which was then undergoing a thorough reorganization. In Erlanger's delightful essay, "A Physiologist Reminisces," he tells with modest dignity and interesting personal detail of his role in the evolving Wisconsin Medical School.[3] Erlanger writes that the attic laboratories at Wisconsin were empty and that the first two years were devoted chiefly to organization. His signal services to Wisconsin included fostering instruction in small groups, stimulation of productive scholarship, and subscription to the major physiological journals as a beginning for the medical library.

His early work in the diagnosis and understanding of heart block and his studies on blood pressure received high praise. Later, in 1914, Erlanger and his younger associate, Herbert Gasser, formerly a student and instructor in physiology here at Wisconsin, were jointly awarded the Nobel Prize for their discoveries regarding the highly differentiated functions of single nerve fibres.

To make the two-year school possible, other appointments followed in rapid succession. Only brief characterizations will be given here; more complete descriptions of the men and their accomplishments will follow as the departments developed.

To help Erlanger with his many tasks, Dr. Harold Cornelius Bradley from Yale was appointed in 1906 as assistant professor of physiological chemistry. He was long and lean, with an all-embracing smile, delighting in the out-of-doors, in university life, and devoted to people. He was born in Oakland, California, in 1878, and spent his early life in Berkeley, where his father was a member of the University of California faculty. He went to Yale to study physiologic chemistry, when that subject was being developed chiefly under Lafayette B. Mendel. In Wisconsin this subject was at first given in the department of physiology, but was soon granted departmental status.

Arthur S. Loevenhart (1878–1929), always ready with a laugh and an amusing and pertinent story for every occasion, came here in 1908 from Johns Hopkins as professor of pharmacology. He was born in Lexington, Kentucky, on December 29, 1878, and had an unusually varied succession of clinical and pharmacologic contacts. He was graduated in medicine at Hopkins in 1903 and at the time he came to Madison was associate professor of pharmacology and physiological chemistry at the older institution.

Another Hopkins graduate, Charles Henry Bunting (1875–1961), grew up roaming the bluffs and studying the wild flowers along the Mississippi River near his home, La Crosse. A graduate of Wisconsin with a fellowship in biology under Birge, he later had superb training in pathology at Hopkins under Welch and at Pennsylvania under Dr. Simon Flexner. Bardeen brought him here in 1908 from the University of Virginia, where he was professor of pathology, to fill the similar chair at Wisconsin.

When Erlanger left for Washington University in 1910, still another Hopkins Medical School graduate, John Augustine English Eyster (1881–1960), cultured Virginia gentleman, son of a physician, and broadly trained, was persuaded to leave the professorship of pharmacology at the University of Virginia to head the department of physiology. His close associate for many years, Walter J. Meek, had come here in 1908 from A. J. Carlson's laboratory at Chicago to help Erlanger in physiology. By 1910, when Eyster became chairman, Meek was assistant professor; he proved thoroughly competent in all phases of the demanding professorial duties; later he became chairman of the department, assistant dean, and during World War II acting dean of the Medical School.

This small group of young idealists, average age thirty-one, formed the nucleus of the faculty for the preclinical years of our attic medical school, as it was dubbed in mild derision because the laboratories were in the attics of Science Hall and the old Chemical Engineering Building. The close quarters threw the men together, aiding in the mutual development of their laboratories and of a splendid spirit of cooperation and devotion to teaching and research. Classes were small; helpful ties with the rest of the University became common. To a large degree these early appointees and their immediate associates set the pattern of teaching, of research, and of deep interest in the University. They placed their stamp on the graduates of the Wisconsin two-year school; the warm loyal allegiance of these students, who had to go elsewhere for most of their clinical training, still continues.[4]

In discussing the beginnings of the two-year Medical School, we must not forget that our clinical departments started with a few young internists whose duties were the care of the health of University students.

As is so commonly the case when a broad, forward-looking step is contemplated, it took a shock — in this case, a tragic one, a severe outbreak of typhoid fever — to produce action. This preventable disease was taking a high death toll throughout our country in the early part of this century, with especially heavy incidence in rural areas. In 1908, about 35,000 deaths were reported. Since the ratio of cases to deaths was approximately tenfold, that figure meant 350,000 cases.

With 5,000 students from different areas, some of which had high typhoid rates, the University could not expect to remain exempt. Early in November, 1908, a student, whose regular work was the wiping and stacking of plates and dishes in a popular boarding house, came down with a gastrointestinal disease that initially received that ancient diagnosis of cholera morbus. Other cases soon broke out among the boarders, and shortly thereafter a diagnosis of typhoid fever was made.

On December 15, 1908, Ravenel, the head of the state hygiene laboratory, wrote to Van Hise that there had been thirty-four cases and three deaths; subsequently there were four more reported deaths, or a total of seven, indicating an epidemic of about seventy cases. Ravenel exonerated the milk supplies, ice, and water. He stated further that the student suspected as the primary case went home on October 31 and died two weeks later. Ravenel continued, "His death blocked further investigation and it will probably never be possible to prove this source of infection. However the exclusion of all other sources of infection points almost certainly to this origin of the outbreak."[5]

As many of the sick students went home, some to their death, the University hygiene committee, with Ravenel as chairman, and the medical faculty strongly urged the appointment of a medical advisor for the University.[6] Erlanger and Bradley, who had been at the University of California in Berkeley where a comprehensive student medical service had originated, were strong supporters of the idea. Dr. Bardeen recognized the importance of the recommendations and that their fulfillment would give an opportunity to appoint to the medical faculty a man well trained in internal medicine.

Prior to this time, Dr. James C. Elsom, director of the men's gymnasium, and Dr. J. Helen Dobson Denniston, director of women's physical education, gave such attention as time and facilities permitted to minor medical problems of the students. Through Dr. Bardeen, who was president of the board of the Madison General Hospital, the Regents had made a rather indefinite arrangement with that institution to admit students when hospital care was needed, with payment of costs for the indigent.[7]

The typhoid epidemic, and an outbreak of diphtheria following closely on its heels, pressed upon the Regents the need for better control of housing and student health. Active discussion arose with strong conflicts of opinion. Opposition to the idea of a University physician developed promptly among some of the local physicians and from broader areas. Dr. John M. Dodson, formerly a prominent physician of Madison and at this time dean of Rush Medical College, representing one phase of the opposition, voiced the strong objection to what was named "contract medicine." Local physicians joined in the cry. Dr. Bardeen responded in a noteworthy letter:

I think the Regents can see as little reason why they should not hire a physician to look after the students at the students' expense any more than they should not put up dormitories for students because it would interfere with the income of keepers of student rooming houses and boarding houses. They look upon the University as a state and not a city institution, and do not feel that the Madison physicians have a right to object on personal financial grounds to measures taken by the Regents for the welfare of the student body. . . .
It seems to me the time is likely to come when most people will insure themselves not only against death and accidents but also against sickness, and the tendency will be for the big insurance companies to look after the health of the person insured against sickness. If this time should come, the physician's duty will be primarily to prevent people's getting sick rather than [as] it is now to be called to help a person out of trouble when he is so far gone that it is difficult to do much for him. . . . The transition will doubtless be hard on many individuals, just as the transition from handmade work to machinery has been hard on many individuals. . . . If there is a transition from the methods of private practice of today to general hospital and contract practice mentioned above, there will doubtless be a loss of that finer personal touch which the best family physicians have with their patients today; and this loss will probably be more than compensated by having greater scientific treatment given to the great mass of individuals.[8]

Bardeen met the "contract medicine" attack directly and with appreciation of the many factors involved:

The only just criticism of contract practice that can be made, as far as I can see it, is the attempt so often made, especially in lodges, to furnish a large amount of medical service for a very small sum. Under such conditions, either very inadequate service can be rendered, or the physician is given a very inadequate return for a large amount of service, and against either of these practices, the medical profession is and should be united.[9]

I believe it is as futile to attempt to block the better kind of contract practice in medicine as it is to try to block the formation of corporations in the business world. We should insist on the highest standards.[10]

University Regent Dr. Edward Evans of La Crosse, president of the State Medical Society, took up the cudgels for a student health program. He marshalled his arguments effectively and persuaded the doubters. A letter to a prominent opponent, Dr. Charles Sheldon of Madison, gives us something of his persuasive methods:

I may say that we have the hearty and cordial support of all the best men in Milwaukee. It is not intended to interfere with any of you there in Madison, any more than every forward move along the line of preventive medicine is bound to curtail our monetary income. Don't grouch! Don't knock! Push! Pull! Nothing else would fit you!! [11]

Many of the objections ceased, including those of Dr. Dodson, when the original plan of charging a special medical fee was dropped. All appointments were to be on the regular faculty basis and additional funds were to be obtained by a slight increase in the regular incidental fee. This had the dual effect of preventing the student from thinking that all medical care could be obtained through the University, as well as placating the fears of local physicians about "contract practice." [12]

After Regent approval of the plan for a medical advisor, Bardeen succeeded in obtaining a man with splendid experience in internal medicine, a broad public-minded point of view, and rare human qualities — Dr. Joseph Spragg Evans. Evans, who had had his medical training in Pennsylvania (M.D., University of Pennsylvania, 1899) and in several European centers, was called to be medical advisor and professor of clinical medicine. With his clinical skill and his personal charm and deep interest both in patients and in friends, he was a key figure, "the heart," in the development of the Medical School. Dr. Evans' diplomatic and friendly approach to Madison helped to alleviate adverse criticism.

Despite objections and unfavorable publicity in the local press, the Wisconsin student health program began its services in February, 1910, in the Cornelius house on State Street next to the corner of Park. The plans for this service and its limitations were well outlined by Bardeen and were approved by the Regents.

The use of the Student Health Service expanded so rapidly that Dr. Robert Van Valzah was appointed in 1910, Dr. William S. Middleton in 1912, and Dr. Frederick Rinker in 1913, a highly effective group of physicians all trained in medicine at the University of Pennsylvania. With later appointments, as the work expanded and the two-year school developed, the student clinic became the nucleus of the department of medicine with responsibility for clinical instruction and patient care. Dr. Evans' tact and the appointment of Drs. Reginald H. Jackson, Thomas W. Tormey, and Joseph Dean as lecturers in clinical medicine relieved, in a measure, the local tensions.

4 World War I
Including the Gas Warfare Unit
at the University of Wisconsin

*Can anything be more ridiculous than that a man should have
the right to kill me because he lives on the other side of the
water, and because his ruler has a quarrel with mine, though
I have none with him?*

Pascal

The normal growth of the Medical School and the University was progressing admirably under the Van Hise–Bardeen re-
gime, when on a summer's day, June 23, 1914, in the small Serbian town
of Sarajevo, a half-demented member of a terrorist organization mur-
dered the Archduke Francis Ferdinand, heir to the Austrian Empire, and
his young wife. There was always trouble in the Balkans, so at first no
one realized that this was the spark that would touch off an overwhelming
world-wide conflagration.

Older alumni will remember that Woodrow Wilson was re-elected
President partly at least through the influence of the widely heralded
slogan, "He kept us out of war." Many factors were part of a gradual
change in attitudes. The war at sea, the loss of ships, lives, and food essential to Britain and Western Europe, the submarine warfare, and the
sinking of the *Lusitania* were powerful influences that turned us against
German ruthlessness. By April, 1917, many, probably most, of our people were ready to vote for war. On April 6, 1917, Congress voted overwhelmingly that a state of war existed with Germany.

Our senator, Robert La Follette, bitterly opposed the war; he was one
of the determined and lonely isolationists. His attitude caused much turmoil of spirit in the faculty of the University. The University faculty
resented La Follette's opposition to the war, and most of us signed a resolution condemning his stand. In Van Hise's words, "When war was de-

clared, on April 6, 1917, there was not an instant's hesitation in the decision of the faculty that the University should participate in carrying the war to its successful conclusion." [1] Intensive military instruction, the change from the two-semester to a three-term routine, the many faculty members, in or out of uniform, who were engaged in war work, the selective service draft for students — all these were immediately or gradually a part of the disruption of normal life on the campus. Many students and faculty members were drawn into the war; those who remained on the campus carried on the local burdens. The meatless days, the wheatless days, and the double-duty classes come to mind as a small part of the war effort.

The University catalogue for 1917–18 gives a brief but excellent statement of the deep impress of the war upon the life of the University. Strong efforts were made to continue the educational work and at the same time to train men for war through the Reserve Officers Training Corps and also at Fort Sheridan.

The plea of Surgeon General Gorgas of the U.S. Army for medical mobilization was met to a high degree, although most medical students were required to continue their professional training.

The introduction of chlorine and other war gases by the Germans caught the United States and her allies quite unprepared. Frantic efforts were made to develop appropriate defenses against gas attack, and it became necessary to organize a broad program. Initially the gas warfare work was handled by a civilian group of the Bureau of Mines under Yandell Henderson, professor of physiology at Yale. During the early part of 1917 the U.S. Army organized the Chemical Warfare Service. Since the biological aspects were particularly important, outstanding pharmacologists were recruited at once. At the University of Wisconsin Medical School, Dr. Loevenhart, well known for his studies in biologic oxidation, was asked to help in the effort, and Dr. Bradley went to Washington in uniform to act as personnel officer in the development of the Chemical Warfare Service.

Some thirty members of the U.S. Army, who had had chemical and biological training, came to Madison to work with Dr. Eyster and Dr. Meek, now Majors in the Army in the Chemical Warfare Service and leaders of the Medical Defense Division at Wisconsin. They studied chlorine gas, phosgene, mustard gas, and lewisite, with dogs as the usual experimental animal. The basement and first-floor laboratory rooms of

Science Hall provided space where gassing chambers were constructed. Records were carefully kept, and detailed studies made on the effects of different concentrations of the several gases. Oxygen therapy was suggested as a promising mode of dealing with respiratory injury from the inhaled gases.

This work continued until January, 1919, when the unit was disbanded. During the first part of 1919, Eyster and Meek wrote a detailed account of the studies that had been made at Wisconsin, but unfortunately this was never published; this illustrated monograph was sent to Washington and because of its secret character was retained in the confidential files of the War Department.[2] Much of this work was repeated later during the early days of World War II.[3] In a brief history of the early work sent to President Birge, the War Department warmly praised the University and the men involved.[4] The following Medical School faculty members were stationed here in Madison and worked actively in these investigations with Major Eyster as the leader: Victor C. Jacobson, Chauncey D. Leake, J. Y. Malone, Walter J. Meek, L. F. Richdorf, Benjamin H. Schlomovitz, and Edwin F. Schneiders. Harold C. Bradley and Arthur S. Loevenhart worked chiefly in Washington in the same service.

This work was the most significant scientific contribution by members of the medical faculty during the war years, although some other small studies were also made. Robert Drane, William F. Lorenz, and William S. Middleton are listed in the 1918–19 catalogue as on leave of absence to engage in war service. They served with distinction in the American Expeditionary Force.

Aside from a few confirmed pacifists and, as always, some who opposed this particular war, the eagerness to serve in some capacity in the war was almost universal. The sensitive attitudes of those whose duties required them to remain at home is well shown in the warm friendly letter from Dr. Evans to his younger colleague, Dr. Middleton, when the latter was returning to this country after the war.

You will find the crowd a bit sensitive over the failure to get into service. As much as I have suffered as the result of disappointed ambitions along that line, I believe that Bob [Van Valzah] and Fred [Rinker] have suffered more. The sacrifices they made to stick by when army service would have given a relief can never be estimated nor repaid. I am older and can stand it better but I regret many times each day my willingness to step aside and allow Lorenz to go with the Wisconsin troops, for the experiences at the Marne would have meant much to me. I realize that Lorenz did the job better than I could have done, but nevertheless, the disappointment is strong.[5]

<h1>5   Beginning of the
Four-Year Medical School</h1>

*The medical and biologic sciences have advanced in these
later years with strides unapproached and in directions
undreamed of but a quarter of a century ago. New vistas of
knowledge and power have been disclosed, the full fruits
of which will be gathered by coming generations. The main
cause of this unparalleled progress in physiology,
pathology, medicine and surgery has been the fruitful
application of the experimental method of research, just
the same method which has been the great lever of all
scientific advance in modern times. Strange as it may seem
at the turning-point of the century we are here, not as we
should be, to ask you to foster and encourage scientific
progress, but to beg you simply not to put legislative
checks in its way.*

William H. Welch in a speech opposing
the anti-animal experimentation bill, U.S. Congress, 1900.

President Van Hise, still urging "nothing less than the
world's greatest university," died shortly after the Armistice, November
11, 1918, and Professor Edward A. Birge was appointed in his stead.
After friendly scar tissue had formed over the tragic personal wounds
from World War I and the disruptions in "life, liberty, and the pursuit of
happiness" had dwindled, the University and the Medical School turned
to the problems of growth that now fell upon them. The veterans returning to take advantage of the Soldiers' Bonus Law of 1919 and the
children that had recently reached college age pushed enrollment from
5,000 to 7,000 by the fall of 1919, and by the first of 1920 to 7,500.[1]
Insufficient staff, buildings, and budget dumped perplexing questions into
the laps of President Birge, the Regents, and the legislature. The high
cost of living and faculty salaries below those of neighboring state uni-

versities became matters of debate in Madison and to a degree throughout the state.

The paramount problem for Bardeen and his faculty was legislative approval of the four-year medical school and a large teaching hospital to make this possible. These were giant steps. Dean Bardeen declared that the Medical School had reached a "critical stage." [2] With 100 students in the second-year class and 150 in the first and with the increasing difficulty of placing two-year graduates in good schools because of restrictions on the number of students in these schools, Bardeen argued that the University had only three choices. It could restrict enrollment, give up the Medical School entirely, or establish the complete four-year course.

In a report to President Birge and the Regents, Bardeen elaborated on these alternatives.

Alternative 1) is impractical if the restriction in numbers is to be made sufficient to make it likely that all worthy students are to be placed in good schools. The limit would have to be 15 to 20 students. There are good reasons for limiting the number of students accepted in a class to 100 or less but a limit so high would not affect the purpose in question.

Alternative 2) is preferable to alternative 1) but should be accepted only after most careful consideration. Nearly one-half of one per-cent of the adult male population belongs to the medical profession. The state laws now require longer and more expensive training for this profession than for any other. If the state is to provide for higher education at all it certainly should for this important branch. While up to now the state has depended on private endowments or public support elsewhere to supply wholly or in part the medical education of those training for the practice of medicine in Wisconsin the increasing cost of medical education is making it constantly more difficult to maintain this parasitic attitude toward this branch of education.

Alternative 3) is in line with the recent policies of the Board of Regents, the State Board of Education, and the State Legislature. All have looked forward to the completion of the four year medical course at the University. It has not hitherto, however, been evident that immediate steps to this end are imperative. If we cannot place our students elsewhere for clinical training we have no right to encourage them to take the first two years of the medical course here. If they are to have better chances to enter medical schools by taking the premedical work at the universities in which those schools are situated we have no right to encourage them to come here for their work. If we enter upon a restrictive attitude of this kind we cannot hope to retain here a medical faculty of the quality needed for Wisconsin standards. If once the medical work thus far established . . . is allowed thus to disintegrate it will be difficult in the future to build it up again. The state cannot permanently get along without support of medical education. To build it from the ground up would be a difficult and expensive proceeding. On the other hand, by establishing a complete medical course Wisconsin will reap many benefits from support of medical education which she now misses. At present far too many of those who receive their premedical and the first half of their medical course at Wisconsin fail to return to the state after completing the medical course elsewhere. The best men are offered attractive opportunities where they graduate. By giving a complete medical course of high standard Wisconsin would insure a continuous supply of well trained physicians for the state.

The University of Wisconsin has taken just pride in service to the state. In one of the most important services which a university can render the state, that of medical service, this university however is far behind the universities of the states which border on Wisconsin. Michigan, Illinois, Iowa and Minnesota have long had complete medical departments, an essential function of which has been the giving of the best of medical care to those who because of poverty would otherwise have had to forego such care. Where this care is offered, a few weeks of treatment furnished by the state may make a productive citizen out of one who might otherwise be a lifelong inmate of a charitable institution. No expenditure of public funds is likely to give greater return than that spent for scientific treatment of disease.[3]

The all-important bill removing the previous two-year restriction and approving a four-year medical course was passed by both houses and approved by Governor Philipp on April 25, 1919.[4]

Our professor of medicine and director of the student health clinic, Dr. Joseph S. Evans, close friend and intimate adviser of President Birge, was sent as unofficial emissary to talk over the problems of the University with Governor Philipp. Almost immediately, Dr. Evans won the Governor's confidence and esteem. Although initially the Governor had taken positions thought to be adverse to the University, he had by this time become aware of its difficulties and sympathetic to its needs. He strongly approved of a single board to control all the state-supported institutions of higher learning, although he was not able to put this plan into effect. Governor Philipp had already called one special session of the legislature to provide the soldiers' bonus. Now Dr. Evans asked him to call another special session to provide a million dollars for the University.

The Governor was finally persuaded to call this session in May, 1920. Adroitly he asked the legislature to consider legislation under which some of the unused balance remaining in the soldiers' bonus fund would be returned to the general fund and then appropriated for the construction of a Wisconsin General Hospital as a memorial to those who served the country in the war. This was a suggestion worthy of a Daniel. With such a proposal before them, the legislators would hardly dare to adjourn. By this means the University would obtain a hospital, and the four-year course that had been approved earlier could be developed.

Following the passage of the bill suggested by Governor Philipp, affairs looked favorable for an immediate advance towards the complete four-year medical school for teaching, research, and state service that Bardeen and Evans had been strongly urging. However, there were obstacles in the path — financial, personal, and political. Typical of repeated troubles are several that occurred prior to the approval of the building of the hospital.

One early stumbling block was the Allen Survey of the University, a voluminous, one-sided study conducted by W. H. Allen of the Bureau of Municipal Research in New York City, and his many aides for the Wisconsin State Board of Public Affairs.[5] This was one of several surveys of state institutions designed to improve their business organization. Van Hise and the faculty promised full cooperation, but Allen became so antagonistic and partisan that the faculty and the press later turned against him. Through his excessive emphasis on cost-accounting methods, he aroused the distrust of the faculty and the administration. One example was his emphasis on the great waste of building space in the University because some of the buildings were not used to capacity for the full day. Faculty committees led by Professor George Sellery of the history department, later dean of the College of Letters and Science, demolished most of Allen's arguments. The highly involved story of the survey, running over several years (1912–15), was summarized by Van Hise in this way: "Its chief conductor, Dr. William H. Allen, was an undoubted annoyance; neither the benefits nor the end effects of his work have been important." [6]

Several years later Birge gave his opinion on the futility of educational surveys: "Insiders failed because they were too much under the control of the traditions of the institution. Outsiders are apt to give too little consideration to these same historical considerations. They criticize the institution as if it were detached from the conditions under which it has grown and which have made it what it is, and their criticisms are very likely to be impracticable for this very reason." [7]

In Allen's brief examination of the Medical School, he queried the adequacy of the two-year school and the high cost per student. Dean Bardeen's rebuttal included statements that our two-year graduates were well received and continued competently in the good schools of the country, and that even with only two years of training our students had proved capable as emergency interns in Madison General Hospital. Finally he quoted the highly regarded Flexner Report of the medical schools of the country which commended our school, but hoped that adequate hospital facilities for the four-year school would be forthcoming.[8]

Another more serious obstacle, as far as the Medical School was concerned, was the bill introduced in the Wisconsin legislature in 1915 by Senator J. H. Bennett of Viroqua. It was typical of several bills that have been introduced from time to time to prevent the growth of the school; these have had considerable support from some of the local physicians. The Bennett bill was originally designed to restrict Medical School teaching to nonclinical subjects; later it was modified to limit the course to two years; and still later, more favorably amended by Bennett himself to permit broad medical services by the University clinic to students.

Bardeen opposed the bill and succeeded in obtaining support for the complete four-year Medical School. Among helpful supporters were Dean Germain of Marquette Medical School and Father Moulinier, also of Marquette; they deplored the evident local interests behind the Bennett bill.[9] A member of the Board of University Regents, Dr. Gilbert F. Seaman, was especially effective in opposition to the amended Bennett bill, which subsequently failed to pass, leaving the development of the two-year Medical School as approved in 1907.

While we were waiting for the political pot to simmer down, during 1916–17, the first two buildings designed specifically for clinical and Medical School purposes were approved, carried through the drawing board stages, and finished by 1920. The sorely needed Student Infirmary, for which we had been striving for so many years, was finally built, paid for partly by an appropriation of $43,000 from the legislature, and by the generous gifts of $25,000 each from fellow Madisonians Carl Johnson and Thomas Brittingham. The other building, the Mary Cornelia Bradley Hospital for the study of children's diseases, was also made possible by gifts from Dr. and Mrs. Harold Bradley and from Mrs. Bradley's parents, Mr. and Mrs. Charles R. Crane, in memory of the Bradley daughter, Mary Cornelia; the University contributed $18,000. These two hospitals were opened in 1919 and 1920 and were used even before they were completed by patients during the great influenza epidemic. These were the first buildings erected specifically for clinical purposes; they helped to scatter the doubts about whether or not a complete medical school could ever be achieved here.

Immediately following the passage of the bill establishing the State of

Wisconsin General Hospital and the appropriation of the necessary funds, Governor Philipp advised the University administration to prepare plans for the hospital at once, to let contracts and begin building before his retirement at the end of 1920. He realized that a change of administration might alter the attitudes towards the hospital and that the prices of construction were continuing to rise.

Orders were given and the state architect's office prepared the plans. Although the complete contracts were not signed, the Regents decided to go ahead with the pouring of the foundation. The last concrete was poured December 20, 1920, but further building was stopped. The foundation lay boarded over for two years while questions of a possible increase in taxes or a deficit in the state treasury were under consideration. Finally in 1922, Governor Blaine, finding that the balance in the soldiers' bonus fund continued to increase, agreed to sign the order for construction. The building then went up with only the usual delays. Patients were admitted in September, 1924.

The first clinical class of twenty-five students was admitted in the fall of 1925. In June, 1927, in the dignified commencement ceremonies, each of the twenty-five students, nineteen men and six women, was escorted to the platform individually by a member of the medical faculty, presented by Dean Bardeen, and appropriately hooded. By vote of the faculty and with the authority of the Regents of the University, President Glenn Frank conferred the first degrees in medicine awarded by our University. It was a simple ceremony, but vitally important, and, may I state, quite moving for many of the faculty, and doubtless too for these first M.D.'s of the University of Wisconsin. It was seventy-nine years from that day in 1848 when the University of Wisconsin was incorporated with a "department of medicine" designated as one of its constituent parts.

THE FIRST CLASS OF THE UNIVERSITY OF WISCONSIN TO GRADUATE WITH THE DEGREE OF MEDICINE, JUNE, 1927

Ruth Anderson
Charles F. Burke
Marie L. Carns
John I. Chorlog
Norman V. De Nosaquo
Myra Emery

John A. Grab
Margaret Hatfield
Vincent Johnson
Everett Keck
Beatrice Lins
Chester Long
Raymond Ludden
Wendell Marsden
Frank Mason
John T. Morrison
Jeannette Munro
Carroll W. Osgood
Burton S. Rathert
Didrik Sannes
Milton Senn
Russell Sterling
Jack Supernaw
Harry Vander Kamp
William Werrell

6 Problems of the Clinical Years

Three faces wears the doctor, when first sought
An angel's, and a god's, the cure half wrought,
But, when the cure complete, he seeks his fee
The devil then looks less terrible than he.
Euricius Cordus, of Erfurt, Germany
First half of the sixteenth century

The surging advances in knowledge during our forty-year period have obviously required continuing alterations in the individual courses of the Medical School. The broad plan of instruction in the first two years has, however, changed but little. The first year is devoted largely to normal anatomy, gross and microscopic both before and after birth, and to physiology, both physical and chemical. The second year considers disease processes, different types of injury, the many causes of injury, including microorganisms, and the reaction of the body to these injuries. Methods of altering these reactions by drugs and other methods are presented. Courses in gross and microscopic examination of the body and the body fluids are an important part of the work in the second year. The third and fourth years take the students more directly to the bedside and the wards where medicine and surgery are paramount, and the many specialties begin to present their peculiar problems. I shall not attempt to consider the many moot questions of curriculum changes that have occupied committees through all the decades or the overwhelming changes after World War II. However, the preceptor plan of Bardeen was a most important change in the curriculum of the fourth year.

In meeting the problems of effective clinical teaching, Dr. Bardeen made a noteworthy contribution to medical education. He realized the value of the close contacts of physician and apprentice in the earlier centuries and he saw that teachers of today in our modern hospitals and laboratories could only partly present to the students the art of medicine, the immediate problems of the physician in competitive practice, and the importance of environmental influences in understanding and treating the patient.

"With your help we are about to try a new experiment in medical education, a combined academic and preceptor system."

Dean Charles R. Bardeen thus introduced the topic of a revival of the time-honored but abandoned medical preceptorship of an earlier generation. The time (November 12, 1926) was propitious for the initiation of any change in clinical instruction, since with the completion of the Wisconsin General Hospital (1924) the first four-year class of the Medical School was entering its senior year. His audience at the hospital on this momentous occasion included the following representative physicians from the state:

> John M. Dodd, Ashland
> H. Christian U. Midelfart, Eau Claire
> Hartwig Stang, Eau Claire
> Adolph Gundersen, La Crosse
> Sigurd Gundersen, La Crosse
> Edward Evans, La Crosse
> Karl W. Doege, Marshfield
> Walter Sexton, Marshfield
> J. B. Vedder, Marshfield
> F. Gregory Connell, Oshkosh
> Neil Andrews, Oshkosh
> Merritt L. Jones, Wausau

As Dean Bardeen enlarged the topic of preceptorships, he said, "We desire to have the medical profession of the state reassume the spirit of responsibility for the training of the coming generation of practitioners and we desire to have our students spend as much of the course as possible in close association with masters of the art of medicine. This is possible only through the re-establishment of preceptor training under modern conditions. On the other hand, we desire to have the student sufficiently grounded in the basic and medical sciences and in the principles of diagnosis and treatment as to be able to take advantage of the privilege of working in close association with a busy master of the art of medicine. . . . You here tonight are, I hope, to form the entering wedge of a gradually broadening movement along these lines."

Thus was launched the Wisconsin Preceptorial Plan that has thrived over the past thirty-seven years. Its conception was the product of Dean Bardeen's fertile brain. Contrary to certain opinions, its genesis was not in the prospect of limited outpatient demands in Madison but on the broad basis of the widening gap between the practice of medicine in a modern university hospital and in the field. His perspicacity becomes more evident with the passage of time. Essential to the fruition of Dean Bardeen's plan was the enlistment

of the support of outstanding clinicians in the state. In this relation and in
the continuity of effort, Dr. Joseph S. Evans, Professor of Clinical Medicine
(later professor of medicine and chairman of the department) played the
major role.

Inherent in any plan of cooperative education are the acceptance of responsibility and the sustained effort of all participants. Such has been the
fortunate lot of the University of Wisconsin in the remarkable fidelity of the
preceptors to their assumed task.[1]

To make the preceptor plan feasible, the fourth year was increased
from thirty-two to forty-eight weeks and was divided into quarters. The
curriculum is now arranged so that each student spends one quarter with
the chosen preceptor. While on this extramural service, each student is
required to write a series of careful case reports which are sent into the
office of the Medical School. In addition, at the end of the service each
student furnishes a written report describing the nature of the service,
telling the main benefits derived, and making suggestions about possible
improvements.

During the year each clinical center in which extramural teaching is
carried on is visited several times by members of the faculty of the Medical School. At the beginning of this work the preceptors-in-charge were
invited to Madison for a conference. In addition, many of the preceptors
visited the University during the year to give lectures before faculty and
students.[2]

In a 1950 survey by Dr. W. S. Middleton we find the following statement: "After twenty-three years of experience in the field of undergraduate medical preceptorial teaching, the Wisconsin verdict is unqualifiedly
in favor of its continuance. . . . The several preceptors took a natural
pride in the opportunities and the development of the young medical
students."[3]

A still later report (1960) on the preceptor program stems from a
four-year study in which the authors have tried to balance the favorable
and unfavorable facts and attitudes. In summary the authors state: "We
believe that in the setting of the University of Wisconsin Medical School,
the preceptor program makes a valuable contribution to the total educational effort." They also cite the 1955 report of the Council on Medical
Education and the Hospitals of the American Medical Association to the
effect that "twenty-four medical schools in the United States offered preceptor programs. These were required in ten schools and elective in the
remainder."[4]

Obviously, our major preceptors and also many of their younger col-

leagues have in the period of these surveys gone through several of the
ages of man; they have played many parts and have played them well.
Some of the earlier men have to our deep regret gone all the way to the
end. I am including a list of preceptors from the 1944–46 catalogue.
Both their grateful students and their colleagues on the faculty in Madison
delight in honoring them.

Preceptors-in-charge, 1926–50

Ashland

John M. Dodd
Frank D. Weeks

Eau Claire

H. Christian U. Midelfart
Peter A. Midelfart
Hartwig M. Stang

La Crosse

Adolph Gundersen
Gunnar Gundersen
Edward Evans
William E. Bannen
Matthew A. McGarty

Janesville

William T. Clark

Marshfield

Karl W. Doege
Walter G. Sexton

Oshkosh

Frank Gregory Connell

Rhinelander

Warner S. Bump

Sheboygan

Paul B. Mason

Wales

R. H. Schmidt, Jr.

Wausau

Joseph Franklin Smith
H. H. Christensen
Joseph Smith
Merritt LaCount Jones

Milwaukee

John Huston
Max J. Fox
Silas M. Evans
Einar Daniels

Another less radical change in teaching the third- and fourth-year students has been the presentation of patients and case reports from the combined point of view of medicine and surgery with the hope of stressing the essentials in the disease picture rather than one that may be confusing through the too early introduction of the specialized points of view. With the many changes in medical practice during the succeeding decades, and the varying personnel, the presentation of this broader point of view has necessarily varied in its effectiveness. Dr. Ovid Meyer, long-time chairman of the department of medicine, states: "In this integrated course for third year students, each subject was discussed concurrently by the several departments concerned. For example, diseases of the thyroid would be discussed by someone from medicine on one day, by the surgeon the next day. Pernicious anemia, as another example, would be fully discussed by the internist and the neurologist in cooperation. This plan, which has appeared to be highly successful, was first suggested to Dr. Bardeen and Dr. Evans by Dr. Middleton."[5]

The use of the terms "full-time," "geographical full-time," and "part-time" — and of the title "clinical professor" to indicate part-time appointments — has plagued all the medical schools of the country, including Wisconsin. Toward the end of the last century, men specially trained in the preclinical sciences were being appointed to medical faculty chairs in these fields. These men devoted their full time to teaching and research, so that commonly new standards of achievement were maintained that busy practitioners, however competent, could not meet. Inevitably, the question arose as to the advisability of similar full-time appoint-

ments to the chairs in medicine and surgery. One of the more persuasive discussions of the highly involved problems was presented in
1902 by Dr. Lewellys F. Barker, at that time professor of anatomy at
Rush Medical College, University of Chicago. He urged the development
of what he termed "real university medical schools" in which the clinical
professors would do no outside practice for personal gain. They were to
receive adequate salaries and all fees earned in their consultation practice would be paid into the common university treasury.[6] Interesting indeed is the fact that in 1913 when Johns Hopkins Medical School was
given funds to try this method on a considerable scale, Dr. Barker, by
this time professor of medicine at Hopkins, was, to his deep regret, unable
because of family commitments to retain the professorship even though
the salary seemed generous for that period.

Many have been the variations on this full-time principle and the
problems have been considered carefully by knowledgeable men of high
ideals with differing answers. Manifestly, conditions vary greatly in each
institution and in the same institution in different decades. A recent
Johns Hopkins Medical School catalogue (1964–65), the institution
where the "full-time" seed was first sown, states that "each of the clinical
departments of the school is now staffed by men and women who devote
their entire time to teaching, hospital practice, and research, as well as
by practicing physicians who perform these duties on a part-time basis."

The University of Chicago catalogue for 1963–64 presents briefly the
position of the "complete full-time" advocates. It states that it "is the
only medical school in the country with a completely full-time clinical
teaching staff. In contrast to the part-time program in which the teacher-
physician maintains a private practice and spends only a fraction of his
time at the school, in the completely full-time program every clinical
teacher devotes all of his time in the University Hospitals to the teaching of the medical students, to the care of the patients, and to medical
research. The teaching of students and the care of patients occur simul-
taneously and are considered to be complementary processes. The constant presence of the clinical teaching staff under the full-time plan provides unusual opportunities for intensive training at the bedside and
for the development of a close teacher-student relationship."

As the University of Wisconsin moved into the problems of the four-
year school during the 1920's, Dean Bardeen realized that he could not
maintain a clinical faculty on the same financial terms as were sufficient to

attract the professor of anatomy or physiology and the faculties of the other colleges of the University. His budget was quite inadequate to attempt a bona fide full-time clinical staff. Quite apart from the greater earning capacity of the clinical men, especially surgeons, under our competitive system, the desirability of a broader clinical experience provided by a well-selected private practice has been repeatedly emphasized. One observes also that the men appreciate the independence derived from a private practice. The full-time clinical men here at Wisconsin were permitted to have private practice provided that "this did not interfere with the teaching or research duties." Always it was recognized that the private cases should be used for teaching purposes. Although this has varied in detail, most private patients in our hospital have through the years served for teaching, the major function of the school. The application of the Bardeen rule depended on many factors, including the dedication and commitments of individual physicians. Understandably, it became a basis of conflict with physicians who paid their own office expenses. In the minds of local physicians, some full-time faculty men have misused their privileges. On the other hand, some of our part-time clinical faculty have given of their services so liberally that only by detailed inspection of the official records could one determine the distinctions between part- and full-time.

When Dr. Middleton became dean in 1935, he immediately faced these difficulties by calling a conference of the clinical faculty. He has summarized the matter in this way:

Perhaps Dean Bardeen did not comprehend or foresee the inevitable friction and alienation of the medical profession, local and statewide. Certainly the State Medical Society had occasion to establish a committee on Medical School Relations that became in effect a grievance committee — and its proceedings related almost exclusively to the competition of our clinicians with other physicians in the state. Naturally this attitude was accentuated in Madison where most of our staff actually maintained offices up town.

With certain convictions in the matter, I had maintained that we would be in a much stronger position were we to confine our professional relations to a consultative or reference practice. On these terms, patients would be seen only in consultation and upon reference of another physician. I held that the dignity and strength of our position would be greatly enhanced — and the opposition would perforce dwindle. . . . In a word we were not subsidized by the University to compete with our fellow physicians. I proposed an immediate discontinuance of competitive practice and a limitation of service to consultation and reference. After a trial of six months, should there be any reservations, the question should be reopened for discussion.

The clinical staff accepted this proposal without a dissenting vote and the ensuing performance was a credit to their good faith. By general agreement, the level of [additional] income was fixed at a figure not to exceed the academic salary. As you may recall, the privilege of private patients in the Hospital was granted on the nomination of the chairman of the department and the vote of the administrative committee of the hospital.[7]

This type of practice on a so-called "full-time" basis has continued throughout the period of our history. Conflicts have continued, but on a decreasing scale. With the rapid changes in our affluent society and extensive growth of other hospitals in Madison with increased cooperation in services and in medical student instruction, the difficulties of competition have, I am happy to say, diminished. Some self-interest is essential in life from the first time the babe is placed at the mother's breast; balancing self-interest with public weal is always difficult. The Medical School needs increasing cooperation among all the physicians of the state and especially with the physicians and hospitals in the Madison area.

We are indeed grateful to the physicians of Madison and the state who in the early days when we were struggling to build up the clinical teaching, came repeatedly to our aid. They served with nominal stipends or none and were accorded various titles. They taught sections in physical diagnosis, served as occasional lecturers, and several Madison physicians, notably Dr. Reginald Jackson, held surgical clinics.

In 1920, two devoted physicians from Milwaukee, Dr. Frederick J. Gaenslen in orthopedic surgery and Dr. G. V. I. Brown in plastic surgery generously agreed to come to Madison one day each week to initiate services and teaching in their respective specialties. They were placed in charge of these important branches of surgery. A few years later, 1925, Dr. Otto H. Foerster, also of Milwaukee, similarly agreed to begin a service in dermatology. It is a pleasure to acknowledge our special debt to these men, each of whom served so admirably on a part-time basis with little return save the knowledge of an important contribution to medicine in Wisconsin. Each was successful in building up an effective service and in training competent younger men to follow him. Few now realize how feeble we were clinically at that date and how little we had to offer.

I am listing those men whose names occur in a succession of University catalogues under the two early departments of medicine and of surgery. These men helped to bridge many gaps and gave help in a difficult day. I am certain that Hippocrates as well as all of our early faculty would express thanks to the following Madison physicians:

Homer M. Carter, Pediatrics
James P. Dean, Surgery
Joseph W. Dean, Surgery
Hugh P. Greeley, Medicine
Carl S. Harper, Obstetrics and Gynecology
James A. Jackson, Surgery
Reginald H. Jackson, Surgery
Harry M. Kay, Medicine
Mark E. Nesbit, Ophthalmology
Wellwood M. Nesbit, Eye, Ear, Nose and Throat
George H. Robbins, Medicine
Edwin F. Schneiders, Obstetrics and Gynecology
Arthur G. Sullivan, Surgery
Eugene S. Sullivan, Surgery
Albert R. Tormey, Surgery
Thomas W. Tormey, Surgery

7 Charles Russell Bardeen

May we now turn back and follow Charles R. Bardeen, the visitor to Madison whom we met in our first chapter. For a while we shall be following chiefly the man rather than the "brain."

Although Bardeen was born at Kalamazoo, Michigan, on February 8, 1871, he passed his boyhood in Syracuse, New York, where his father was a teacher. After a year in the Teichmann School in Leipzig, Germany,[1] he entered Harvard in 1889, graduating in 1893, the year the young medical school at Johns Hopkins University was breaking with custom and establishing vastly higher requirements. He was admitted to the first class, and four years later, by alphabetical chance, he was the first person to receive the M.D. degree from the institution.

An undated letter to his father written while he was still a student at Johns Hopkins Medical School provides us with an introduction to the idealistic side of a man whom few knew intimately; it also stresses what all persons with long professional training regret — the seemingly excessive period of economic dependence. The content of the letter leads me to think that it was written during the depression years, probably 1894–95.

Baltimore
Thursday

My dear father,

It seems to me that the only real happiness of existence is that derived from working for those one loves and with those one loves toward a common

41

purpose. The purpose is not of so much account (though some definite end must be aimed at in all exertions); but the sympathy of unity of work is all important. One feels the need of putting one's forces into union with the efforts of others or with the more or less personified and idealized "forces of nature," or more commonly both, in order to get the peace of mind which one feels most worthy of attainment; the peace of mind the Christian feels — the brotherhood of Jesus, and that which Dante felt in the fight "with God" against the evil about him.

The trouble with a life of preparation, of long education, is that all is preparatory to future co-operative effort and all exertion is spent on a pretty narrow self. In the belief that as a physician I should be most useful as a member of society, I thought it best to accept your support if you could afford it and to live a narrow life of preparation in hopes of a broader life of activity. But as I have written you before, I have felt that I was losing much in being supported when I could support. And so it was with a degree of exultation that I read your letter this afternoon. At last an opportunity to work for those I love and who have done so much for me. I shall still look forward to sometime seeing my way to the chosen profession but I far prefer standing by you in the thick of the battle of life, to drifting into the fame of a Hippocrates supported by you until I struck a fat professorship.

Your affectionate son,
C. R. Bardeen

We know that Bardeen did not leave medical school, so we may assume that financial conditions in the family improved.

The next glimpse we have is that of the young Bardeen so competent while he was still working for his medical degree that Dr. Mall recommended his appointment as an assistant in anatomy; despite some opposition in the faculty, Mall had his way.[2] Bardeen continued his teaching and research at Hopkins until 1904 when President Van Hise persuaded him, at the age of thirty-three, to become professor and chairman of the department of anatomy at a salary of three thousand dollars.

This appointment changed his life from one that had been largely devoted to research with some teaching to one that also included increasing administrative duties and complex public relations. Another vital change was his marriage in 1905 to the artistic Althea Harmer, who presided so graciously over his home until her untimely death in 1920. Her talent for generous hospitality made their home a welcome center for acquaintances and friends.

A series of her letters to her father — some eighty of them, but all undated — extending through most of her life here in Madison give welcome, homely glimpses of Charles as a father, of his pleasure in entertaining guests in the home, and of his interest in carpentry and golf; they also reveal a man, who, although devoted to his family to a high degree, generally kept his own counsel. Since letters give so much that more formal comments obscure, I am quoting directly from a few of these letters.[3]

Charles came home this noon with an old winter hat under his arm and a new straw on his head and announced the Medical bill and University appropriation had passed the Assembly 60 to 14. The president appreciates what Charles had done and has made it known very generally that the favorable action was due to his aggressive activity. It almost slumped at one time and Charles gathered all his forces together with strenuous advice, including the president. The president, realizing mistakes had been made, acted nobly and generously. Charles says he is a big man with high ideals, but no politician. I told Charles I thought it took a trickster for that — but he has proved that it can be done with organizing power.

The family elation over the passage of the bill approving the two-year medical school gives further color to the official story as vividly described in Curti and Carstensen.[4]

A more personal letter gives a delightful picture of the charm of Helen, their young daughter.

She is bewitching now. Charles makes more fuss over her than he has with either of the boys. He tried his best to hold back, affecting a scorn for girls, but she was too much for him. She is precocious about doing things, pulls herself to her feet and many other things which Charles refused to believe until he saw for himself. He then admitted it was remarkable.

A later letter tells of the older boys, William and John, and the early capacity of John in mathematics.

William and John are both entering the University High School. John is three years under age but he is what the boys call a "cracker jack" in his studies as well as in his games.
Charles asked William why John did better in football. William replied, "John just hangs on and won't let go." He does the same thing in his studies. When he comes across anything difficult he puts up a big fight.

Much later, in 1956, John was awarded the Nobel Prize jointly with William Shockley and Walter Hauser for their investigations on semiconductors and the discovery of the transistor effect.

A story about Bardeen that was bandied about in Mendota Court, where he lived with his family, amused us all. Workmen who were busy laying concrete sidewalks were bothered by Bardeen's sons and some of the neighbor children, and Dr. Bardeen gave the boys a sharp reprimand. Whereupon one of the neighbor mothers said, "Why, Dr. Bardeen, I thought you liked children." He responded promptly, but in his accustomed somewhat mumbled fashion, "I like 'em in the abstract, but not in the concrete."

All sources emphasize Bardeen's persistence and energy; his work week included Sundays, although he did take time off for golf. His son William tells the following characteristic stories.[5]

As soon as his feet touched the floor in the morning, Bardeen would roll a Bull Durham cigarette — and a feeble, wobbly, invertebrate cigarette it was. Tobacco was all over his shirt and on the floor; but the limp cigarette hanging out of the corner of his mouth did provide a few puffs.

Bardeen also typified the absent-minded professor. After automobiles became relatively common, Dr. Bardeen used his considerably to go to the golf club. One day he drove back from the club and stopped at the drugstore where he commonly bought his tobacco and his cigars. Coming out of the drugstore, he walked home. Later, he wanted to take the family for a ride, and the car was not in the garage. Great excitement! He called the police and said, "My car's been stolen." The police came and, of course, found the car where Bardeen had left it.

William also remembers being taken to Science Hall on Sundays and wandering around the dissecting rooms. Dr. Bardeen usually went in at the tower door, the northwest door, where there was a hand-operated elevator — a great delight for the children.

Dr. Bardeen was unquestionably the most important man in the up-building of the Wisconsin Medical School. Over many years he was the dominant but not the domineering figure. He was keenly intellectual, self-assured, strongly independent, with broad interests and high ideals of scholarship. He represented, as did all the early members of the Johns Hopkins Medical School, the ideals of a university in the German sense, one in which research and scholarship were the major interests.

He was not a magnetic personality, not readily responsive; he did not draw men to him as did Dr. Joseph Evans. He followed his determined path and expected each person to choose and follow his own. In the early period, University policy commonly assumed that responsibility for administrative decisions rested to a high degree with the deans and the president. We had faculty meetings at the end of each semester to make the promotion of students legal and executive committee meetings, comprised of the chairmen of the departments, somewhat more frequently. Occasionally a student would be voted out by the faculty and then would turn up back in class — decision of the dean. But this seemingly troubled the faculty very little. Bardeen supported the decisions of each faculty member, even when he obviously doubted their wisdom, and the faculty in turn supported the decisions of the dean. I remember asking Bardeen why certain general problems were not brought up for faculty discussion. He responded that the final decision was his, so why take the time of the faculty. Dr. Bardeen spoke in a somewhat mumbling fashion, moving his lips only slightly, but he thought with clarity and there was no mumbling in his decisions.

Dr. Bardeen was a prodigious worker, a patient, tolerant man, simple in his tastes, keenly intellectual, with continuing aspirations for a strong productive department of anatomy and similarly for a medical center that would influence favorably every section of the state. He was a reserved man and persevering almost to stubbornness. Although there were, quite naturally, differences among the faculty and between the faculty and Bardeen, the faculty and the dean worked well together for the common purposes of the Medical School and the University. As Walter Sullivan has said of Bardeen, "Recognizing no particular creed, he antagonized none." [6] Bardeen enjoyed people and the pleasure of entertaining them in his home. His conversation and queries showed the wide range of his interests. In the anatomy department, also, the relationships between Dr. Bardeen and his associates were relaxed and friendly.

As one reviews the development of the Medical School and the serious opposition that Bardeen sometimes had to face, one is impressed with the calm way in which he met the difficulties and with his persistence in achieving desired ends, with emotions under excellent control. He may have been boiling inside, but outwardly he remained calm, marshalling his facts and gathering advocates for his cause from far and near.

Bardeen's philosophy of faculty appointments was, "Do not buy big names, but choose young men of promise." With a few exceptions, subsequent history showed that his judgment about these growth possibilities was sound. In his teaching philosophy, Bardeen tended to follow his mentor Dr. Mall, but he was more interested in teaching than was Mall, who represented the German university point of view more completely with emphasis on research and on placing the student entirely on his own feet. Bardeen commonly chose good teachers as his younger assistants and also for the more permanent faculty of the department. Even in the later years, when he was heavily involved in administrative duties, he usually gave the final oral examinations that all students approached with "fear and trembling."

His teaching methods can best be recalled by citing letters from students and faculty. From Dr. Richard TeLinde, long-time professor of gynecology at Johns Hopkins Medical School, come the following illuminating letters:

Five of us came from Wisconsin to Hopkins during World War I at the time of the great flu epidemic. I remember so well that the Wisconsin contingent (with the exception of the writer) always stood out very prominently when a question of anatomy was asked. I must confess that the Hopkins boys were not too strong in that subject. Often the question would go around the class and finally be answered by one of the Wisconsin contingent. It got to be so that whenever one of the Wisconsin crowd would answer a question in anatomy correctly the usual remark was, "Oh well, of course, he studied anatomy at Wisconsin." [7]

I too admired Bardeen and his organization of the medical school; however, I do not believe that he was a great anatomy teacher. The students had very little contact with him until examination time. Then we approached him with fear and trembling. We had not learned our anatomy from him. We learned it from the instructors who were in the dissecting rooms and held Saturday morning quiz sections. In these quiz sections, we quizzed the instructors as much as they quizzed us, and cleared up many points which were confusing to us. Bardeen claimed to be a follower of Mall's conception of teaching and he himself practiced it, but fortunately his staff did not conduct itself along that line. The instructors gave us a great deal of individual attention and really taught. I remember particularly John Skavlem who was clear headed and a wonderful teacher.

It seems to me that absentee teaching offers a wonderful excuse for the professor who is either so engrossed in his research that he doesn't want to "waste" his time teaching or who is too lazy to teach. [8]

From Dr. John Skavlem, formerly associate professor of anatomy, University of Cincinnati, now in private practice, come the following comments.

Dr. Charles Bardeen was thought of and spoken of as "Chuck Bardeen" among his medical students. This appellation on the part of students did not in any sense imply a feeling of undue familiarity with him. He was once and always Dean, and Professor, with all the respect, admiration, and recognition of authority which such positions commanded. It was felt and recognized that the administration and control of the medical school gained its strong direction from the office of Dean Bardeen.

The course in human anatomy as he gave it had no didactic lectures. Dr. Bardeen at the beginning of the course held a "convocation" in which he impressed on the student the seriousness, the respect and dignity that must be recognized in dissecting a human body. "You are privileged to be operating on a fellow human individual." After such introduction to the anatomy laboratories you were privileged to choose pretty much your own dissecting partners, advised to buy an anatomy text, assigned a cadaver and allowed to proceed at your own pace.[9]

Dr. Hance F. Haney, professor of medicine, University of Oregon, tells an amusing anecdote:

An incident that stands out vividly was an anatomy oral final examination on head and neck. This examination was taken by a group including about ten other classmates — one, a capable girl. To our surprise, in walked Dr. Bardeen. All we knew about him was that he was Dean and that he asked rather demanding questions. The first question, as I recall, was directed at me as follows: "What is the function of the head?" After several attempts, Dr. Bardeen drew a planarian on the blackboard and located on the head two sensory organs, and it became obvious that the answer wanted was that the function of the head which is common to all animals that have a head, is that it enables the organism to become aware of objects at a distance. The next question was directed to H. F.: "Mr. F., if you met a pretty girl walking down the street, what nerves would you use?" H. colored a bit and found himself virtually unable to utter a word and the question was carried on around the group with somewhat similar responses. On the second round Dean Bardeen said, "Mr. F., you would wink at her, wouldn't you?" This of course was merely the leading question in getting into the details on the extrinsic muscles of the eye, their innervation including all the pathways concerned between the retina and those muscles. Shortly thereafter in walked a little black and white spotted terrier named Peter. Peter was grouchy to the extent that if one tried to pet him he would usually take a snap at the would-be friend, and all of us respected him. Nevertheless, he came in wagging his tail. Dr. Bardeen asked our girl classmate, "Miss O'S., what can that little dog do that you can't?" She snapped back, "Wag his tail, Dr. Bardeen." Dr. Bardeen then cleared his throat and said, "That's right," and went on to the next question. There was not the slightest smile on his or any student's face.[10]

A letter from one of Dr. Bardeen's close anatomy department associates, Dr. Harland Mossman, is especially appreciative and illuminating.

I would not say that he was not an effective teacher, for in his informal, often blundering way, in lectures and laboratory, he succeeded in directing students to the understanding of essentials, and I am sure stimulated them by his obvious interest in the subject, but more especially by his interest in them as human beings.

I lived in a state of almost daily surprise and sometimes shock or in what still appears to me as righteous indignation over the casualness and tolerance in the conduct of the courses and the handling of students in the anatomy department. However, I soon became convinced that the basic principle of treating students as adults and allowing them to manage their own affairs was far better than the system in which I had been trained in the zoology department. I must say without delay that the great majority of students responded to the friendly and tolerant attitude of the faculty and were better students, and I am sure became better men in later life than they would have become under a more regimented system.

His grading of the lab books for his course in embryology, a part of the work of the students during the semester, was a revelation. On the day of the final examination, Dr. Bardeen wrote questions on the little portable blackboard, sat down behind a table at the front of the room and asked for the lab notebooks. They were brought up, around 120, most neatly bound in black thesis covers. He rolled a cigarette, and then started "grading" notebooks. He would look at the title page, which seemed best when it contained the title of the course, the year, and Dean Charles R. Bardeen as professor. He would then flip through the rest of the pages in less time than it takes to tell it and put down a grade. Well-bound books with the proper title page, small, noncommital, but neatly colored drawings, and a neat black-lined border around each page rated an "A." Lesser degrees of perfection suffered accordingly.

I had the temerity to contrast his grades with mine, which had been worked out carefully, and to point out numerous extreme discrepancies to him. His reply was, "Isn't it interesting how close I can come to the correct estimate of their work by the rather quick look I take at their notebooks?" I was speechless. His grades stood.

He liked to draw with colored chalk and would have the little 4′ × 7′ portable blackboard smeared in no time, and himself likewise, as he would erase with his bare hand or sleeve, drop chalk on his vest and wipe the sweat from his face with his chalky hands. By 9 o'clock he would stalk out, reminding one of a Pawnee in war paint.

Dr. Bardeen thoroughly enjoyed teaching, especially in the laboratory. His pertinent questions of distinctly unconventional type aroused the curiousity of the students. Of course the students kept a record through the years of these unusual questions and could obtain a high grade without knowing much about anatomy. Had our grading in gross anatomy depended upon his examinations, there would have been complete chaos.[11]

Dr. Bardeen's scientific publications, comprising about a hundred titles, show the breadth of his interests and also the high quality of his detailed studies. We find historical essays such as "Anatomy in America," and "Physicians Through the Ages," as well as reviews of anatomical texts and papers that might well be classed under sociology. One of his early works (1897–99) that is still cited, described the visceral changes in extensive superficial burns and also in fatal burns.[12] He was one of the earliest students of the effect of X-rays on living cells such as amphibian ova; he noted the variation in susceptibility at different stages of development (1909).[13] His continued use of X-ray studies on living subjects helped to keep anatomy alive for his students. He first proposed determining the size of the heart from its X-ray silhouette, a method that still has clinical use.[14] His detailed study, "The height-weight index of build in relation to linear and volumetric proportions and the surface area of the body during post-natal development," published in the *Contributions to Embryology* by the Carnegie Institution of Washington (1920), is regarded as one of his most scholarly contributions. His formulae for heart size, growth, and build, and his simple mechanical analysis of muscles are also highly regarded.

Judging from his frequent mention of his studies on planaria, we may assume that these were among his favorite publications. In a letter to his friend, Dr. Yates of Milwaukee, written a few years before his death, Bardeen stated, "Wisely or unwisely, I have permitted my public interests to interfere with my scientific work to the serious detriment of the latter." As we review Bardeen's scientific achievements and his public service to medicine and to the state, we realize how much he accomplished in both areas.

Dr. Bardeen also showed strong interest in community affairs. When he came here, he found that Madison was far below the accepted minimum for a community of its size and character in hospital beds and in hospital service standards. He soon became president of the Madison General Hospital board, and both he and Dr. Bradley were active in the campaign to increase the membership in the association. Their efforts, added to those of the community, were successful and in 1912 the desired new wing was built. Following Dr. Bardeen, E. J. B. Schubring became president and pushed the continuing growth of the city hospital. Throughout those early years, this hospital was an important resource for the University. The hospital accepted student patients, and the Regents arranged to reimburse the hospital for the few who were indigent. In that early period some local suspicion, and indeed active opposition, to the idea of the University Medical School prevailed, but this has gradually subsided. Following Dr. Bardeen, Dr. Walter Sullivan and later Dr. Otto Mortensen, also of the anatomy department, became members of the Madison General Hospital board. Considerable mutual appreciation has developed, especially through the instruction of their student nurses by members of our faculty and by the instruction of our medical students in several surgical and medical services in the hospital, as well as by the service of our graduates as interns.

Also, when Bardeen came here, no central gathering place existed where faculty members from the widely scattered departments could meet for discussion and entertainment. He was one of a small group that organized the University Club and purchased the Parkinson property for such purposes at the corner of State and Murray streets. The present, much-enlarged University Club has served these and other functions and has weathered many financial storms.

Bardeen's diverse interests came to a focus on the Medical School and the problems of medical education. His contributions to medical education were considered earlier when we discussed the rapid development of the clinical departments after the building of Wisconsin General Hospital.

<h1>8   Joseph Spragg Evans</h1>

Medicine is learned at the bedside and not in the classroom.
William Osler

Joseph Spragg Evans, the "heart" of our Medical School [1] and the man all the early clinicians delighted in calling "the chief," was born in West Chester, Pennsylvania, on March 6, 1875, the only son of the Reverend Joseph S. and Ruth A. Evans. The morning paper of West Chester on Friday, June 26, 1891, sheds light on the young Evans. He was the salutatorian of his class in high school and gave an oration with the title, "Stimulus of Opposition." His opening sentence was, "There is a great deal of truth in the saying, 'Kites rise against, not with, the winds.'" Almost two decades later, as the University historians, Curti and Carstensen, showed, Dr. Evans did indeed meet strong headwinds here at Wisconsin and rose successfully against them: "Only a man of Evans' fiber could have weathered the vicious attacks from all quarters made on the student health service immediately after its initiation, attacks, which, stimulated for obvious reasons by certain local doctors, recurred at intervals throughout the years." [2]

Returning to the young Evans, we find that he went on from high school to Haverford College, was graduated in 1895, and earned his medical degree in 1899 from the University of Pennsylvania. After a six months' houseship at Germantown Hospital and sixteen months at the Hospital of the University of Pennsylvania, Dr. Evans had the opportunity, so highly desired at that period, of a year of further study in Berlin, Vienna, and Paris. In Vienna he was happy to have the opportunity to work with Weichselbaum in bacteriology, and in Paris, he studied briefly at the Pasteur Institute under Metchnikoff. On his return to Philadelphia in 1902, he began the private practice of medicine and continued

51

his academic pursuits as instructor in clinical medicine in the University of Pennsylvania School of Medicine. He also had an associateship in the William Pepper Laboratory of Clinical Medicine from 1902 to 1909.

The story of a serious epidemic of typhoid fever among the students at the University of Wisconsin, the consequent recommendations of the University committee on hygiene, and the decision of the Regents that a medical advisor was essential for the University has been told earlier. After considerable local and state opposition to the proposed plan, Dr. Joseph Evans was chosen; he came to Madison in February of 1910 to be the head of the Student Health Service and was given the title of medical advisor and professor of clinical medicine.[3] After the Medical School became a full four-year school in 1924, Dr. Evans received the title of professor of medicine and continued in that position until his retirement in 1945. Whereas Dr. Bardeen left behind him innumerable reports and letters for the record, Dr. Evans left few letters and few published papers, but innumerable admiring warm friends, including each patient and almost all persons with whom he came in contact. He worked wonders through these personal contacts like another earlier Philadelphian in other fields, Benjamin Franklin.

We shall now visit a while with Dr. Evans, chiefly through a number of his friends. Dr. Middleton has written:

In the broadest sense of the term, Dr. Evans was a medical statesman. Possessed of a charming personality, he dominated every gathering to which he lent his presence by his easy grace and gentility. Kindly and gentle by nature, his indomitable courage and steadfastness to high medical ideals vigorously resisted and overcame apparently insuperable obstacles to medical development in the Middle West. His inherent kindliness, which pervaded every sickroom upon which he was attendant, brought untold comfort to the afflicted. His wise counsel was sought by people in all strata in society and his sympathetic ear was open to the humble as well as to the mighty.[4]

A story of Dr. Evans under fire shows another side of the man. The workers at the city laundries went on strike, and the conference with the officials and the labor groups included Dr. Buerki, Dr. Evans, Dr. Stovall, and Dr. Middleton. As one would expect, Dr. Buerki led off and talked a great deal. Finally, the chief, Dr. Evans, made a strong plea with regard to the necessity of clean and sterile linen for patients and for women in labor. He declared to the conference, "I shall crucify you if a single woman dies or some serious accident occurs because of your failure to provide us with clean linen." He carried the day with strong language, and the laundry said that they would see to it that the hospital was not injured by the strike.[5]

A letter from Dr. William Oatway provides a lively description of Dr. Evans and his methods:

Dr. Evans was an ideal administrator, a fine medical manager, and a great arranger. The "ideal administrator" delegates authority quite well, and Dr. Evans searched and connived and persuaded in order to get the personnel to do the various medical jobs. He then let them do their work with a minimum of guidance and no interference at all. Dr. Evans had been a fine clinician in his early years at Wisconsin, but after his twenty-five or thirty years of administration, he jokingly would say, "A physician must know his patients; he must know to whom they should be sent for special care; and he then doesn't have to know much detailed medicine."

During the development of the Medical School and the coincidental construction of the hospital and the school buildings, Dr. Evans proceeded in a way which could be described by terms used in later years as "operating" and "finagling," and he loved it. He liked to let a situation develop by way of the influence of friends, patients, time, necessity, political contact, indebtedness, etc. He then would wrap up the solution to the problem by a happy combination of circumstances and a half-hour conversation at the right time with the right person.

He liked the use of his full name, "Dr. Joseph Spragg Evans," when it was used in a formal way. He was usually called "Dr. Evans" by those who were not close to him, "Dr. Joe," by older friends and patients. He was proud to be referred to as "chief" by his staff. He was "Uncle Joe" to his family and close friends, and to a large circle of contacts and admirers who wouldn't think of saying it to him in person.

His professorial duties during the years just before and just after 1920 consisted chiefly of a small group of lectures on physical diagnosis. These were formal, not as exciting as we had expected, but well supplemented by the practical section work in the long-gone red brick student health clinic on Langdon Street. Dr. Middleton always insisted that the student squeeze every bit of information out of his eyes, hands, and stethoscope before being helped by x-rays, etc. This was perfectly proper and correct, Dr. Evans agreed, but with the stipulation that if a person depended on a physical examination alone "he had better drop his stethoscope out the window," since it could do more harm than good.

Dr. William Pepper of the University of Pennsylvania Medical School and Dr. Evans gradually formed a habit of meeting once a year after Dr. Evans had gone to Wisconsin. They could then discuss and agree on the Wisconsin two-year students who would be transferred to Pennsylvania for the final two years. The mode of selection and acceptance was never well understood, but it seemed to consist of a few conversations with Wisconsin faculty members; no special discussion with the candidates; a selection not always based on scholarship; and a choice of five or six members of the second-year class, usually including one woman. I can well remember being told by a colleague, "You are on the list for Pennsylvania," and saying in disbelief, "I can't make it and no one has asked me." The reply was, "Oh, you'll make it; Dr. Joe has

you on his list." When the notice of acceptance came, it was in the form of
a brief apology from Dr. Evans: "You will have to forego belonging to the
first four-year class at Wisconsin — I have promised you to Pennsylvania."
And Elsom, Ritchie, Sander, Packard, Pratt, and Oatway all said, "Yes, sir.
Thank you, Dr. Evans."

Dr. Evans used a mixture of praise and various types of stimulation to
produce the results he wanted from members of his classes and faculty. A
series of quotations, pulled out of the haze of memory, would include the
following:

"I'll save G. B. from the results of this examination; he's too good to lose.
Then I'll take the skin off his lower back and he'll never slip again."

"I gave R. J. a pat on the back; he deserved it and he needed it."

"I called H. B. a scared cat and he'll hate me for years. I was partly right,
but I had to get him to fight back."

"You are giving J. P. his oral examination. He is a favorite of mine. Give
him the toughest oral he has ever had."

"K. P. is the best contact with the lawmakers that the Medical School
has ever had. He gives them the care they need; he does it quickly; he likes to
do it; and they'll remember it forever."

"The preceptor plan is unique and wonderful. I approve and support
and take care of it, but Dr. Bardeen was its source and sponsor and don't ever
forget it."

Dr. Evans liked people — active, interesting people more than others.
He put academic standing second to other qualifications more than once.
He had strong opinions on a great variety of subjects, some of them of no
great importance, but sometimes flattering to his friends. A young physician
and amateur sculptor was making a portrait bust of Dr. Evans, who thought
that certain parts of the likeness were outstanding, and he said so many times.
One of his comments about this topic was, "Bill, when Bardeen gave you a hundred in anatomy, it may have been because you did well and pleased him at the
time; however, when I look at the way you carved the area around my eyes
on the clay bust, I think you deserved the hundred; anybody can see that I
wear nose-pincher eye-glasses!" [6]

Jackman Pyre (M.D., Wisconsin, 1937) was an admiring younger
friend of Dr. Evans during the years "Uncle Joe" lived with the Pyre
family. The sidelights Jack Pyre provides us give a vivid picture of Dr.
Evans at home.

Uncle Joe gave fastidous attention to the correct china when he was
entertaining the "Town and Gown" society for their rotating dinners. The
correct wine glasses, the correct wines, were most important. The meal was
served at our house on occasions and was attended by various dignitaries, only
a few of whose names I remember. I saw them through a crack in the door,
having sneaked downstairs in pajamas to observe. Another memory is of the
barrel of oysters that he got on two occasions and kept in the basement. He
fed them corn meal and we went down to listen to the oysters sucking up
their repast.

He devoted especial attention to each medical student, picking the student's internship for him. I remember his sending H. P., who was a fairly raw country boy from Lancaster, to Dr. Madison and Dr. Squires in Milwaukee. He found that H. P. had never worn and didn't own a hat, so he took him down town, and, I think, bought him one the day before he left for the big city.

He enjoyed the preceptorship trips throughout the state, which he usually took in a rather zippy automobile — at first, the open Cadillac and later the Stutz, the Chandler, and other sporty cars. I drove him as a 17 or 18 year-old on some of those trips, going to Milwaukee, Wausau, Ashland, and La Crosse. Drs. Dodd, Gunnar Gundersen, and Merritt Jones were close personal friends who welcomed his visits.

Visiting faculty from Milwaukee came to Madison regularly and lectured to us at the Medical School. Uncle Joe and I lived in an apartment on Lathrop Drive, and Otto Foerster came each Friday for his lecture and stayed with us. I served them breakfast of shirred eggs. We had a problem with Uncle Joe's expensive hand-towels, since Otto insisted on wiping his razor blade on a hand-towel instead of on tissue. Mother, who took care of the linen, finally gave Otto the same slashed towel each time, but it never occurred to Otto that the cuts were those that he had administered.

Uncle Joe was most particular in his dress — his suits were dark blue, always with a pin stripe. His ties had to be blue with polka dots, and the polka dots had to be one size only. We all made efforts at buying him a different pattern, but they never got worn.[7]

This is such a sharp contrast with Dr. Bardeen's complete ignoring of the matter of dress!

Physicians who were close to Dr. Evans both personally and professionally and with whom I have considered him, his life, and his work, all tell the same story.[8] It was Dr. Evans' warm interest in the patient and his personal problems that endeared him to each one. It was the art of medicine, the medical priest that bound them all to him. Whether it was Senator La Follette, Governor Philipp, or a forlorn, unknown student, all who met him were won by his gift of understanding. He had an uncanny memory for names and faces; he prided himself on this gift. In talking with those who have been his patients, one is deeply impressed with their devotion to Dr. Evans and their understanding of his fidelity to them and their needs and of his willingness to make efforts far beyond the call of professional duty to be of service to them.

This is not to minimize his medical acumen. In consultation on the wards, we recall that at times when the staff was floundering in a diagnostic impasse, Dr. Evans' quiet question, "Have you thought of this?" would not infrequently lead to a correct diagnosis. He seemed to be an intuitive diagnostician. His students recall his deep interest in and his vivid descriptions of the different forms of nephritis. His annual lecture in this field was an event.

A remark by President Birge, a grateful patient and devoted friend of Dr. Evans over many years, suggests what Birge considered a conspicuous difference between Evans and other excellent physicians: "Dr. Evans was able to put himself *inside* the patient."

As a sample of Evans' continuing interest in his former students, Miss Birge writes:

He kept a map during World War II on which he placed the substance of the frequent reports of the movements of the 44th General Hospital. I got my news of their shipwreck and Edward's [Birge's grandson] wound from Dr. Evans because he was thoughtful enough to call me to his office and read me Dr. Weston's letter. His comforting remark was "Don't forget there are more good surgeons out there than at home now." [9]

Dr. Evans wrote few papers. He preferred to work personally and was so successful in his immediate contacts, both social and medical, that increasingly he became the preferred physician of other physicians and also of prominent persons throughout the state. He was called in consultation over wide areas. In his early years, after his European studies, he was deeply interested in the bacteriology of infectious diseases, especially influenza, with emphasis on the bacillus of Pfeiffer, at that time considered the probable causative agent of the disease. Later, he became interested in focal infections as underlying factors in arthritis and diseases of obscure origin. He accepted with considerable enthusiasm Dr. E. C. Rosenow's inadequately established theory of elective localization and wrote a summary on focal infections for *Tice's System of Medicine*.[10] A considerable unpublished paper, "Some diseases of the kidneys," [11] merits comment, as does his interest in cardiovascular diseases.

In the development of the clinical instruction at Wisconsin, he repeatedly stressed the importance of treating the patient rather than the particular disease and he urged the minimizing of departmental boundaries in giving a single combined course in medicine and surgery. In a talk of long ago that Dr. Evans gave to a Medical School Convocation on the art of medicine, he closed with the following sentences.

In addition to accurate knowledge of the science of medicine, it is necessary for a real physician to increase his breadth of intellectual interests, his sympathy with the technique of human relationships. He must be a psychologist, he must be a sociologist, he must avoid professional commercialization, and he must have a love for humanity. Few men possess all of these attributes ideally, but all entering the profession should seek to attain them in the Art of Medicine.

Of course, Dr. Evans had his peccadillos. I can remember instances of strong words, and especially later in life, when crossed, he did fly off. These reactions merely brought him down to human levels, and were always more than counterbalanced by his generosity and selflessness. He did have difficult personal problems. To our deep sorrow, his last illness (1948) in our hospital was due to severe, prolonged cardiovascular disease. He loved us and we loved him.

9   William Shainline Middleton

This fourteenth-century description of the Clerk of Oxenford gives us a splendid picture of Dr. Middleton as professor of medicine. Your author's family knows from direct experience the deep interest and skill with which as a physician he meets the personal and medical problems of his patients. In the broader demands of the teaching hospital, Dr. Middleton's capacity for keen analysis, accurate diagnosis, and human appreciation have been a wonderful stimulus to students and colleagues. To his intimates, Middleton frequently ascribes these qualities to the example and teaching of his medical godfather, Dr. David Riesman, with whom he was house officer years ago at Blockley Hospital, Philadelphia; but to bring forth such excellent fruit, we are all aware that the seed must fall on fertile ground. Furthermore, these descriptions omit a highly important asset — the vigor, zeal, and forthright optimism with which Dr. Middleton has attacked each problem, whether it was competing in his favorite sport, handball, investigating a difficult case, or resolving conflicting opinions in the faculty or among physicians of the state after he became dean of our Medical School.

Dr. Middleton was born in Norristown, Pennsylvania, January 7, 1890. After his medical training at the University of Pennsylvania (M.D., 1911) and a year at Philadelphia General Hospital, Middleton joined Dr. Evans and the Student Health Service in 1912. Save for leaves of absence during the two world wars, Dr. Middleton has devoted himself to medicine and to medical education here at the University of Wisconsin through most of his life. He rose to be professor of medicine in 1933, and in 1935, after the death of Dean Bardeen, he became dean of the Medical School.

As the second dean of the University of Wisconsin Medical School, 1935–55, Dr. Middleton showed imaginative vision, assured decisiveness, and the same persistent determination as his predecessor. He did have, however, a somewhat larger admixture of the "democratic dogma" than Dr. Bardeen. Difficult decisions had to be made, faculty appointments considered and confirmed. That he was able to carry the double load of the deanship and that of an active teacher in the classroom and on the wards showed a remarkable capacity to arrange and to use the hours of his long day.

After Dr. Middleton accepted the deanship at the hand of President Glenn Frank, he remained professor of medicine each day until noon. Punctually at twelve o'clock he marched down the corridor of 4 North in a starched, immaculate white coat, with energetic gait and erect carriage. Having just completed an arduous morning of rounds on the medical wards, involving his vivid bedside teaching to students, interns, and residents and usually also including a number of consultations throughout the hospital, he was ready to take a brief break. In his right hand he grasped a bottle of milk. He then entered his office, closed the door, and apparently partook of his luncheon before going to another office and beginning his duties as dean of the Medical School.[1] By budgeting his time and making careful but ready decisions, he found it possible to handle both jobs with remarkable success.

Promptness both in thought and act was ingrained in Middleton's being. I sometimes thought that he kept his watch a minute fast because at meetings scheduled for any hour, he not infrequently started them slightly before the assigned time. At the end of his afternoon work as dean, he would rush over to the handball courts, and with John Parks and Mead Burke against Middleton and McCarter, join in a rough competitive work-out. By evening, after dinner, he was ready for a long period with the books and journals and facile pen. He loved books and reading; what gift can be more enriching? Over the years he has built up a splendid library in medicine and in broader fields of learning. His papers cover an exceptionally wide range of medical subjects and medical history, including his early essays on the effect of college sports on the heart, many papers on infectious diseases such as tuberculosis, pneumonia or the zoonoses, and studies on cardiovascular diseases and hematologic disorders, such as the confusing anemias. Responding to my persistent requests that he name a few of his favorite papers among his numerous intellectual offspring (some 270 titles),[2] he listed about half a dozen of which I have chosen three written in different decades. One was a variation on the method of palpating the spleen, one with W. H. Oatway, on that unruly member, the tongue — a typical Hippocratic approach to disease — and still another on Hodgkin's disease, for many years one of the major interests of Dr. Bunting and the department of pathology.[3]

Dr. Middleton was devoted to the Miller medical history seminar and study of medical history. For this seminar he wrote many papers; he still continues his contributions in this field. Many of his historical papers cluster around his beloved Philadelphia and the men that made that area a leading medical center. The Medical School Class of 1935 on their thirtieth anniversary reprinted and bound some seventeen of his essays in medical history, choosing several tied in with the history of our school and with the University of Pennsylvania — a splendid tribute.

Dr. Middleton's far-seeing vision is well shown by many examples; one thinks immediately of the small beginnings leading toward the dramatic, spacious medical library, built largely through gifts from loyal alumni. The recognition of the importance of medical history, with a chair in that field, and the McArdle cancer laboratories, are also indicative of his foresight.

When Dean Middleton went off to serve in World War II, Dr. Walter Meek, who had had long experience as assistant and associate dean, was appointed acting dean of the Medical School. Despite the added difficulties because of the war, Dr. Meek filled the position well for the duration. The faculty stood steadfastly by him, and Dr. Coon was especially helpful in the hospital decisions.

Personally, Dr. Middleton is generous and loyal and devoted to his many friends both in this and in other countries. He never forgets a friend, especially when trouble is in the offing, and remembers each student and his whereabouts in the world. He has been greatly admired and a little feared by his students. All will remember, at times with chuckles, and at times with red faces, when a particularly dull response has drawn incisive correction and the questionable privilege of wearing the renowned brown derby until some other student has earned that onus by making a similar egregious error. Dr. Middleton required an erect stance when reports were being given and never never never any hands in pockets. A breach of that bit of student etiquette opened the vial of scorn so that rarely was there a second slip. He soon knew each student in the class, his foibles and even his dating habits. He gave colorful nicknames to many of the students, some of these so pertinent that they have tended to stick long after student days. We recall with pleasure "Bull," "Touchy," "Big Shot," "Powder Puff," "Pushover," and others. This habit lessened many teacher-student tensions.

A story that Dr. Middleton tells on himself stems from a fine third-year student from Argentina, several decades ago. Each student was given a patient and two hours in which to do a complete history and physical examination. As Dr. Middleton was coming back down the hall after half an hour, C. V. stepped out of the patient's room, indicating that he had finished. Dr. Middleton then stated severely that after years of medical practice it took him at least one and a half hours to complete such a task. C. V. looked at Dr. Middleton, bowed formally from the waist, and said, "I must be good, no?" Whereupon Dr. Middleton also bowed formally and continued down the corridor. The incident was closed.

One of Dr. Middleton's talents that continues to amaze us all is the ability to deliver a long discourse on an involved medical subject before well-informed audiences, citing chapter, verse, and dates without a single note. These speeches are always well organized, indicating careful preparation and a remarkable memory.

With the return of Dean Middleton from World War II in 1945, the Medical School took on new life. The overwhelming growth — industrial, intellectual, and in population — new appointments, and striking changes in the climate of discovery, with increased governmental spending, wrought tremendous changes in our lives, and there is no end. The influence of Dean Middleton was felt in the activities of each department; the informed reader will remember in private intimate portions of the history that never can be written. Much of this era is beyond our period and requires a younger pen.

Of course, even deans have their peccadillos, doubtless more conspicuous because of their lightning rod position. Dr. Middleton has an amusing aversion to bow ties and moustaches and, on the other hand, a strong predilection for handsome shoes, well shined. In this day of many cocktail parties, it is appropriate to remark that Dr. Middleton is a total abstainer. Obviously he believes that "wine is a mocker and strong drink is raging." He has never prescribed any alcoholic beverage for a patient.

He has described to his friends some gay parties during the wars, but never even under the pressure of farewells and airplane deaths has he accepted the cup or the bottle. We salute him as a convinced practicing Puritan.

Dr. William Shainline Middleton received an exceptional number of well-merited honors. Although commonly I am not including such lists that are readily available in directories, the *Festschrift* to Dr. Middleton, published in 1964 by the Wisconsin State Medical Society, must be included even though it appeared more than a decade after our terminal date. This beautiful tribute includes appreciative letters and papers from his students and friends, a statement of many honors, his remarkably broad bibliography, glimpses of his assured optimism, and a pungent warning article from his own heart and mind, "Let's give the hospital back to the patients." [4]

Of the triumvirate of forceful leaders in the University of Wisconsin Medical School during our period, Dr. Bardeen, as has been already noted, was well characterized as the "head" and Dr. Evans as the "heart" of the young school. Our third leader, Dr. Middleton, built well on the foundations laid down in the earlier years. He added to the faculty and the curriculum in areas that could hardly have been considered in the leaner years when only the necessities were paramount. Throughout his life in Wisconsin, Dr. Middleton was primarily the teacher-clinician, with complete devotion to the Medical School and all persons associated with the school. [5]

10 State Laboratory of Hygiene

*Public health is purchasable. Within natural limitations
a community can determine its own death-rate.*

Hermann M. Biggs

Physicians and students of today have almost forgotten the tremendous effects of the development of bacteriology in the Victorian era and its further applications in the twentieth century which have so changed our death rates. We know what public health practices have been largely responsible for the changes, especially the decreased mortality rates from infectious diseases. From England earlier, and a few years later in this country, especially from Massachusetts, the public health movement spread. Cities and states established laboratories, frequently in a vacant basement room or attic, to apply some of the diagnostic aids and to study the sources and modes of infection and possible prevention.

In Wisconsin the physicians were prodding our State Board of Health for recognition of these aids. In 1903, Harry Luman Russell and his friend Dr. Cornelius A. Harper, who had recently been appointed to the State Board of Health by Governor Robert La Follette, persuaded the legislature to include funds for the "establishment and maintenance of a hygienic laboratory in connection with existing bacteriological laboratories; and its use, as far as necessary and as arranged satisfactorily to the Regents, shall be given to the State Board of Health."[1] The Regents adopted the rules set up by Harper, Russell, and Secretary Wingate of the Board of Health and named Russell as director of the laboratory which formally opened on October 1, 1903. The University provided a basement room in the new Agriculture Hall along with heat, light, and water. The laboratory could thus take advantage of the existing facilities and would supplement the premedical curriculum then in progress under Professor Birge. The services of the laboratory were open to all health officers and physicians of the state.

Some minor appropriation difficulties arose in the next few years, but by 1907 the members of the Board of Health agreed that the laboratory should remain at the University, and the Regents continued to provide the special allotment in the University budget for the hygienic laboratory. In that year also, Russell became dean of the College of Agriculture and could no longer carry on the duties of the State Laboratory of Hygiene or his teaching. To fill these needs, Dr. Mazyck P. Ravenel of the Pennsylvania State Livestock Sanitary Board was brought here to be director of the State Laboratory of Hygiene and to teach medical bacteriology. While in Pennsylvania, he had confirmed the earlier observations of Theobald Smith, demonstrating the cultural differences between tubercle bacilli from human and bovine sources and the greater virulence of the bovine type for the available experimental animals, especially guinea pigs and rabbits. On the basis of experiment and observation, he and his associates maintained the pathogenicity of the bovine tubercle bacilli for man, especially in the early years of life.

Always sharp in argument, Ravenel delighted in taking issue with Koch, who had earlier maintained the identity of the tubercle bacilli from cattle and from man. Fortunate in having such a potent adversary as Koch in the heated conflict, Ravenel enjoyed the contest and continued to emphasize the issues until the battle was won.

Under Ravenel's vigorous leadership the volume of work increased greatly. An epidemic of rabies in 1909 put a heavier load on the laboratory with the necessity of examining more brains of dogs for the specific Negri bodies and the provision of the Pasteur vaccination treatment for those bitten by rabid animals. The United States Public Health Service provided the vaccine and a local physician employed by the State Board of Health gave the injections. Ravenel's failure to appreciate the rights of others almost ruined the important cooperation between the State Board of Health and the University in the work and support of the hygienic laboratory. Ravenel was gracious and pleasant socially, but he was highly contentious. Both on the campus and at the State Board of Health he had conflicts that resulted in his resignation in 1914 to accept a position at the University of Missouri, where he remained through the rest of his active life. He was the energetic editor of the journal of the American Public Health Association from 1924 to 1941.

With the departure of Ravenel, Dr. W. D. Stovall, who had come here early that year from Tulane Medical School to assist Ravenel, took over the conduct of the laboratory and in 1918 was made director. Where Ravenel was aggressive and contentious, Dr. Stovall was appreciative of the other fellow and skillful at bringing opposing forces together. In a few years the physicians of the state were calling on Bill Stovall for advice.

In the laboratory, also, Dr. Stovall created a friendly atmosphere. As the staff grew, he gave each member the opportunity to specialize, resulting in a sense of individual achievement as well as improved skills and services. When desirable, he sent members of the staff to other laboratories to learn improved procedures and techniques. He says of himself that, even though at times he was engulfed in administrative problems, he always spent some hours each day at the bench so that he kept in touch with the work and the members of the staff.[2]

The chemical studies of the laboratory, such as the analyses of potable water commonly required at that early period, were carried on by the chemist, E. J. Tully. In 1916, M. Starr Nichols succeeded Tully and continued with increasing rank and responsibilities in the laboratory well beyond our history period. He became Stovall's competent associate in many branches of the work. He earned a Ph.D. in physiological chemistry at Wisconsin in 1926 and became professor of sanitary chemistry in 1940. Nichols' investigations included several on the chlorination of swimming pool water and factors in the control of bacteria in these important public recreation facilities. He has also written several fine chapters for a standard textbook on the quality and the laboratory examination of natural waters.[3]

The following statement from the university catalogue of 1930–31 gives some idea of the development of the laboratory; the statement has varied slightly through the decades and has indicated the gradual improvement in space, first to second floor of Agriculture Hall, then to the top floor of South Hall, and then to the excellent laboratories in the Service Memorial Institutes.

STATE LABORATORY OF HYGIENE
W. D. Stovall, Director, Professor of Hygiene

The State Laboratory of Hygiene, located in the Service Memorial Institutes building on the University campus, is at once a University laboratory and the central laboratory for the State Board of Health. The staff is occupied in teaching, in the development of laboratory tests which are of assistance in the diagnosis and control of communicable diseases, in other laboratory procedures with which sanitary science is concerned, and in special investigation.

Last year 54,481 specimens for the diagnosis of diphtheria, typhoid fever, anthrax, rabies, tuberculosis, whooping cough, and other diseases were received from physicians, health officers, public health nurses, and others throughout the state. The facilities of the laboratory are used by three-fourths of the physicians in the state. Prophylactic vaccines are distributed free from the laboratory, and silver nitrate ampules are prepared for free distribution by the State Board of Health.

For the convenience of physicians and health officers, cooperative laboratories have been established in Beloit, Green Bay, Kenosha, Oshkosh, Rhinelander, Superior, and Wausau. The state contributes a portion of the funds required for the operation of each of these laboratories, and the respective cities supply the remainder. These branch laboratories are under the supervision of the director of the State Laboratory of Hygiene, acting for the State Board of Health.

The principal work of both the central and the branch laboratories is in the development and improvement of procedures and new methods for diagnosing, preventing, and controlling communicable diseases, and in the dissemination of information of this sort into every community of the state, thereby directly or indirectly touching the welfare of every citizen.

Increasingly with the changing times the laboratory has offered microscopic examination of tissues for malignant growth and other morbid processes.[4] Following the announcement by Papanicolaou in 1943 about the utilization of cytological techniques for the diagnosis of carcinoma of the cervix, the laboratory gradually made that service available. With the personnel changes in the Psychiatric Institute, the hygienic laboratory took over the Wassermann and similar reactions for the diagnosis of syphilis and certain blood chemistry tests that had been so admirably developed by Dr. William Lorenz, the broad-visioned head of the Psychiatric Institute.

Changes in medical practice and changes in the world at large have modified the needs and the functions of the State Laboratory of Hygiene. Realizing that such developments should be met by appropriate coordination of the several state agencies involved, the legislature in 1949 passed the following controlling regulations:

The state laboratory of hygiene shall be operated to furnish a complete laboratory service to the state board of health for the purpose of administering the rules and regulations of said board and the health laws of the state and to make available to the University of Wisconsin and the state board of health such facilities for teaching in the field of public health as may be derived from such a laboratory.

For the purpose of co-ordination between the state board of health and the university board of regents and for the purpose of determining policies, an administrative committee for the state laboratory of hygiene is created to be composed of the president of the university, the dean of the medical school, the president of the state board of health, the secretary of the state board of health, and the director of the laboratory or their representatives. The board of regents of the university, upon the recommendation of the dean of the medical school with the administrative committee approving, shall appoint the director of the laboratory and such other members of its professional staff as are required for the administration of duties of the laboratory. The technical staff and other employees necessary to the administration of the laboratory shall be employed by the director from the eligibility rolls of the department of administration.

Through the years with the increasing demands on the young growing Medical School, Dr. Stovall has been called upon to fill an astounding number of different positions. From the early twenties he was in charge of the course in clinical laboratory diagnosis for second-year medical students. It was designed to bring together the varied offerings of the several earlier courses and focus the attention of the students on the possible clinical applications of these modes of studying cases. When the State of Wisconsin General Hospital was opened in 1924, Dr. Stovall assumed the direction of similar work in the clinical laboratories of the hospital.

In the early years of the hospital, Dr. Stovall frequently joined Dr. Buerki on his trips through the state so that he came to know most of the physicians and also the county judges who ruled on the indigence of the patients. In 1938, Dr. Buerki, the superintendent of the hospital, was invited by the American Medical Association to serve as director of the study on graduate medical education. Again Dr. Stovall added to his many duties by becoming the acting superintendent of the hospital for the duration of Buerki's leave of absence (1938–40).

Still another of Stovall's achievements was the organization of the somewhat loosely associated courses for medical technicians, which he and Dr. Bradley brought together under the general direction of Alice Thorngate.

Dr. Stovall's investigative studies have quite naturally followed the needs of the laboratory for improved methods and for a better understanding of the underlying questions in the many tests offered. His name appears as a prominent author in some fifty papers published from the laboratory. Of these, we can mention only a few: a study of diphtheria carriers, a paper on undulant fever, one on various fungi, and another on "Vi" antigens in typhoid bacilli.[5]

Stovall's influence with the physicians of the state and his position in medical organizations, including county, state, and the American Medical Association, deserve recognition. As a member, and later chairman, of the State Board of Public Welfare, he was instrumental in planning for the Diagnostic Center and its erection on the University of Wisconsin campus. This branch of the public welfare services has been filling many serious gaps in the diagnosis of difficult cases among our young people.

One more example of Stovall's breadth of interest may be found at Prairie du Chien, Wisconsin. There, in 1833, William Beaumont, a United States Army surgeon, had seized the chance opportunity to study gastric digestion in a young French Canadian, Alexis St. Martin, who had been accidentally shot in the abdomen. The story of Beaumont's persistence and his brilliant experiments has been told again and again. Here where much of his work was carried out stands a museum to honor this pioneer American physiologist. This was made possible in part through the zeal and interest of Dr. Stovall working with the State Medical Society.

When Dr. Stovall reached the official retirement age, the Medical School found itself in such need of his services that he was kept on as special assistant to the dean. Despite personal adversities, Dr. Stovall continues to meet his duties with assurance and with his characteristic charm and zealous optimism.[6]

Again, we must go beyond our terminal date for this history to mention that in October, 1961, the State Medical Society and Dr. Stovall's many friends devoted an issue of the *Wisconsin Medical Journal* as a *Festschrift* to Dr. Stovall. In 1964, the Alumni presented Dr. Stovall with the Emeritus Faculty Award.

11 The Student Health Service and the Early Department of Medicine

*Life is short, art long, occasion brief, experience fallacious,
judgment difficult; but treatment after thought is proper
and profitable.*

Hippocrates

The all-important department of medicine has through most of our period included many of the specialties that by the end of the thirties had developed approved specialty boards. As we go on, we shall use specific subheadings whether each specialty has been given departmental status or not; the distinction is largely budgetary.

In our story of the young and growing Medical School, we have already discussed the beginning of the Student Health Service after the typhoid epidemic of 1908, the bringing of Dr. Evans as medical advisor and professor of clinical medicine, and how the student clinic became the nucleus of the early department of medicine with responsibility for clinical instruction and patient care. As each student in need of medical attention felt the warm personal approach that Dr. Evans always showed, the Student Health Service grew rapidly. Almost immediately, more physicians were needed and added to the staff: Dr. Robert Van Valzah came in 1910; Dr. Sarah I. Morris in 1911; Dr. William S. Middleton in 1912; and Dr. Frederick C. Rinker in 1913. What a splendid staff they were — young, cooperative, enthusiastic, idealistic physicians.

Dr. Van Valzah was born in a small community, Spring Mills, in central Pennsylvania, November 11, 1882. He was the third physician in direct line in his family, and, with a single interruption, this tradition had continued for five generations in America. He was graduated from Princeton (A.B., 1904), obtained his early medical training at the Uni-

69

versity of Pennsylvania, and received his degree in 1908. He had internships and residencies in St. Christopher's and the Hospital of the University of Pennsylvania from 1908 to 1910. He was indeed a splendid physician, with skill, knowledge, and human interest; he left a deep impression upon this University's service.

He advanced regularly from an instructor to a professor of medicine in 1918. As Dr. Evans became heavily involved in broader University and state affairs, Dr. Van Valzah threw his energies into the department and ultimately had complete supervision of the Student Health Service. He continued until 1935 when family affairs took him to a large farm on the great bend of the Potomac in Virginia. With the hope that he might return to the University, he was granted an official leave of absence until his death on November 23, 1946.

Most significant of Dr. Van Valzah's eminent qualities was his bedside manner. A most compassionate physician, he brought into the sick-room a calm reserve and complete command of every situation. His patience and sincerity won the confidence of all of his patients. He was the personification of the best in clinical medicine of this period. An intuitive diagnostician, his brilliant diagnoses were frequently, and remain, the source of amazement to his associates. He was universally respected and widely sought as a consultant. The finest of all tributes to a medical man, namely that of family physician to doctors, was his by eminent qualifications. Hundreds of Wisconsin graduates and faculty members will cherish his memory as a devoted physician and hundreds of his students will bear the stamp of his unexcelled clinical approach in their professional careers.[1]

Of his published papers, Dr. Van Valzah especially liked one based on medical examinations of more than five thousand students and a comparison of their infectious disease histories before entering the University and during residence.[2] In the University, those students who had come from rural areas commonly had a higher incidence of the particular communicable disease prevalent that year than did those that came from the cities. The influence of previous rural life was shown especially among the Short Course students of the College of Agriculture, practically all of whom came from such districts. These students, representing about 10 per cent of the total student body, had about 30 per cent incidence of the current epidemic. Manifestly, much of this difference was due to a specific immunity among the "city dwellers" as a result of previous contact with that disease. Dr. Van Valzah advanced the hypothesis that there were other nonspecific and little understood elements in resistance resulting from life in larger communities. This nonspecific resistance hypothesis was further supported in his detailed report on the 1918–19 epidemic of influenza in the University. Larger series by others in several army cantonments gave additional support.[3] These observations dating from the 1910–19 period are early suggestions of the importance of factors described during recent decades — substances such as properdin, adrenal-cortical hormones, and steroids that are now recognized elements in nonspecific resistance.

Without a University hospital and with only a small infirmary and a smaller budget, the opportunities for advancement in clinical medicine here in the early years were meager, so that most of the younger men soon left for private practice or for better facilities in other institutions. We can name only the few who stayed long enough to meet our time requirement.

Dr. Sarah I. Morris came here from the Woman's Medical College of Pennsylvania in 1911, and continued until 1933, working closely with Dr. Evans and devoting herself effectively to the medical and personal problems of the women students. Dr. Frederick C. Rinker, a splendid clinician, was highly important in the Student Health Service. During the influenza epidemic he was a tower of strength along with Dr. Van Valzah. To our regret, Dr. Rinker left us in 1919 for private practice in his home state of Virginia. Dr. George Hiram Robbins came here in 1917; he was a graduate of Rush Medical College and was advanced to the position of assistant professor before he left in 1927 for private practice here in Madison. While on the staff, he was especially active in the student clinic and in teaching the course in clinical laboratory diagnosis. Dr. William S. Middleton, to the great benefit of the Medical School, the medical profession, and all of his many students and friends, has remained with us since 1912, with interims for war experience and the needs of the Veterans Administration, well beyond the age of official retirement. We have tried in an earlier chapter to describe the man and his distinguished services when, following the death of Dr. Bardeen in 1935, he was named dean of our Medical School.

The overwhelming world-wide influenza pandemic of 1918–19 came inevitably to our campus population, placing a most serious test on the Student Health Service. World War I was still killing and maiming our young men, and our University was struggling on under war conditions with many students under military control in S.A.T.C. and others as applicants for induction.

According to Dr. Van Valzah's detailed report of June 19, 1919, sporadic cases of influenza began to appear early in October of 1918 in one of the military sections and spread rapidly through the campus. As it became imperative to secure more hospital space to care for the crowds of sick students, many of them in uniform, approval was granted by the U.S. General Staff to lease the University Club as an infirmary. "The building was converted into a temporary hospital, was furnished, equipped, and receiving patients within twenty-four hours after authorization to lease." Our medical staff with Dr. Van Valzah as the head, Dr. Frederick C. Rinker as resident physician, and Mrs. Rinker, as wonderfully competent head nurse, soon had the new infirmary in running order. In handling the students in the armed services, confusion resulted because of the conflict of University classes, military authority, and medical judgment. Actually, because of class and social contacts, the medical problem was obviously that of a single group including all students. At the height of the epidemic when available space was at a minimum, a number of the citizens of Madison opened their homes and received convalescent patients in order to make room in the infirmaries for new cases. Volunteer nursing help was supplied by the women of Madison. Temporary infirmaries were established in the top floors of Barnard and Lathrop Halls, where the lower floors were being used as barracks. Van Valzah wrote to Birge, "We believe that no seriously ill case lacked competent nursing and practically every desperately ill case had a special nurse both night and day."[4]

We should not forget that the 1918–19 pandemic of influenza was one of the great disease disasters of world history. Jordan, in his history of that disease, states that, "The total world mortality in the influenza pandemic of 1918–19 can never be exactly known."[5] In many lands, only estimates are possible, with the total death losses probably over 22,000,000. The estimate of deaths for India alone is 12,500,000; the more exact figure for the United States was 548,452 or 527 per 100,000 population. The impact of the disease on our University can be appreciated somewhat by quoting from letters by Bardeen and the report of President Birge to the Regents. Dr. Charles Bardeen, in writing to Colonel Seaman, Regent, serving in the Medical Corps in France, December 12, 1918, commented on the epidemic and the S.A.T.C.:

In my last letter to you, I told you about the S.A.T.C. and also the epidemic at the University.

The S.A.T.C. is now being disbanded and we are all happy over this since it has proved a sad mistake. Men cannot easily serve two masters. With military authorities conscientiously trying to make officers out of a group of men and University teachers trying to conduct University work, the students have been "between the devil and the deep blue sea."

In the Regents' Reports, 1918–20, the President stated:

The University went through two severe epidemics of influenza; the first in 1918, involving nearly 1600 cases (besides those in Section B of the S.A.T.C.) and 48 deaths; the second in 1920, with over 1600 cases but only 11 deaths. No similar epidemics either in their extent or in the number of fatal cases have ever been recorded in the history of the University, and it may be hoped that there will be no recurrence of such calamities.

Dr. Bardeen, in the Regents' Report, 1918–20, wrote:

In Section A, the rapid spread of the epidemic occurred between October 1 and October 15. A period of severe complications followed in about 10% of those stricken with the disease. There were 30 deaths of men students during the first semester, about 1% of the total number registered. There were 3 deaths among the women students, about .17% of the total number.

The Student Health Service has continued under different directors throughout our period and beyond, with varying degree of student acceptance, but rarely with the enthusiasm of the Dr. Evans' period. After the opening of the Wisconsin General Hospital, dual appointments with the department of medicine were usual. The following physicians have served as directors from the beginning in 1910:

Dr. Joseph S. Evans	1910–23
Dr. William A. Mowry	1923–37
Dr. Llewellyn R. Cole	1937–48
Dr. John W. Brown	1948–54

Dr. William Atwood Mowry (1880–1949), a native of Illinois, received his medical degree from Northwestern Medical School in 1909. After a variety of clinical and administrative services, he was brought here by Dr. Evans to take over the direction of student health in 1923. Not too happy in this type of work, he became the first head of the allergy clinic in 1933. This service developed rapidly, but Dr. Mowry always managed to have time for personal teaching of the students and residents. He was a highly sociable person with warm interest in mankind and in varied human contacts rather than in scholarly problems. To his colleagues, he was a friend, ever ready to be of service. We deeply regret his sudden passing on January 8, 1949.

In the allergy clinic, Dr. Mowry was faithfully assisted by Dr. Helen Pratt Davis, who after two years of medicine at Wisconsin, completed her studies for the M.D. degree at the University of Pennsylvania in 1927. Following several years in private practice and in our Student Health Service, Dr. Davis joined Dr. Mowry in 1941 and aided in the care of hundreds of patients each week.

Dr. Llewellyn Rathbun Cole (1902–48) was the highly colorful head of the Student Health Service from 1937 to his early death in 1948. He was a native of Wisconsin who took both his undergraduate and his medical degrees here, followed by a residency in the University of Pennsylvania Hospital. Immediately thereafter, he was appointed assistant physician in student health and in medicine, and proceeded to advance to the directorship of the Student Health Service in 1937 and full professorship in 1939. We probably tend to think too much of Dr. Cole's mannerisms as he wrapped his white coat tightly around his slender body or cocked his head on one side as he got off some pungent remark, but he did a fine job of improving the student clinic. His public health broadcasts attracted much attention and gave opportunity for the display of his wit and his historical point of view. He helped to develop the special clinics for graduate medical education.

Always behind the several heads of the Student Health Service and their rapidly changing staff, Dr. John E. Bentley, as assistant and associate director from 1936 until beyond our period, was the competent physician constantly there, save for the years of war service. For many years he was physician to the athletic teams and enjoyed traveling with them. He was important in training the new men in the clinic. He joined the Emeriti in 1963.

Dr. John W. Brown came to us in 1948 from the department of medicine of the University of California Medical School and four years of service as chief of hospital in the U.S. Marine Corps. He was an especially well-trained physician with broad appreciation of public health problems, and an awareness of the importance of sharply specific diagnosis in infectious diseases in order to use antibiotics more accurately. Infectious mononucleosis and acute hepatitis were among his special interests.[6] Under his leadership, the Student Health Service made distinct advance; preventive medicine was combined with this service and given departmental recognition. Unfortunately, in 1954 ill health forced Dr. Brown's resignation.

12 Department of Anatomy

In the great felicity of this age — which the gods desire to be controlled by your sagacious Majesty — with all studies greatly revitalized, anatomy has begun to raise its head from profound gloom, so that it may be said without contradiction that it seems almost to have recovered its ancient brilliance in some universities; and with nothing more urgently desired than that knowledge of the parts of the human body be recovered, I, aroused by the example of so many distinguished men, decided to give what assistance I could and by those means at my command. And lest all others should successfully accomplish something for the sake of our common studies while I alone remain idle, and lest I achieve less than my ancestors, I decided that this branch of natural philosophy ought to be recalled from the region of the dead. If it does not attain a fuller development among us than ever before or elsewhere among the early professors of dissection, at least it may reach such a point that one can assert without shame that the present science of anatomy is comparable to that of the ancients and that in our age nothing has been so degraded and then wholly restored as anatomy.

Andreas Vesalius

We first met Dr. Charles R. Bardeen as he arrived in Madison back in 1904 to meet with President Charles R. Van Hise. The announced objective of that visit was to see what might be done with meager facilities and less money to establish a productive department of human anatomy. However, the major objective, not mentioned publicly at that time, was the founding of a new medical school at the University of Wisconsin. We have been following Bardeen through two decades and over many blocking difficulties as the Medical School was conceived, was born, and grew up. In this continuing story we expect to follow both a chronological and a departmental order. We shall now consider the first department to be established, anatomy.

Although from the point of view of rank, Dr. Bardeen was the first professor of anatomy, Dr. William Snow Miller antedated him here by twelve years and was the one who first welcomed him during his preliminary inspection trips. During this earlier period, Miller had been on the staff of the department of zoology, teaching vertebrate anatomy, histology, and embryology, especially to those enrolled in the premedical course. From the success of these students as they passed on to several medical schools and from our later contacts with Dr. Miller, we are certain that nicety of technique, accuracy of observation, and thoroughness were well drilled into his students.

William Snow Miller was born at Stirling, Massachusetts, on March 29, 1858, the son of the Reverend William and Harriet Emily Snow Miller. With the foundation of his education in this cultured home, he continued his studies at Williston Academy at Easthampton, Massachusetts. Following a preceptorship under Dr. C. H. Hubbard of Essex, Connecticut, he entered Yale Medical School, graduating in 1879. After a period there as instructor under Benjamin Silliman, he practiced medicine for several years, but then returned to life in the laboratory because of a long illness and a developing deafness which became his great tribulation. For a while he was pathologist of the hospitals in Worcester, Massachusetts, and then from 1890–92 he was a fellow at Clark University. There, under the influence of the anatomist, Franklin P. Mall, he began the study of the lung, a field he greatly enriched throughout the rest of his long life. He was appointed instructor in biology at Wisconsin by Professor Edward A. Birge in 1892.

After the establishment of the Medical School, Dr. Miller, except for a one-year leave of absence in Leipzig and two years at Johns Hopkins, spent much of his active life in charge of the course in histology. In addition to his good teaching, he enjoyed many years of persistent microscopic study on the anatomy of the lung. His noteworthy results were published in 1937 in a long-awaited, scholarly monograph, *The Lung*.[1] It was a best seller; the first printing, 1500 copies, was sold out in a fortnight. A new edition came from the press ten years later, in 1947.

Another splendid achievement of Dr. Miller was the gathering, with painstaking zeal and good judgment over long years, of a valuable medical history library. It was a labor of love. He was well versed in all the classics in anatomy and, to a lesser degree, in other fields of medicine, and his fine library reflected these interests. After his death the University purchased his library to become a cherished portion of our own medical history collection.

Another example of his deep interest in the history of medicine may be found in the William Snow Miller medical history seminar. In 1909 he invited a group of students to join him informally in his rooms at the University Club to consider some of the great names and achievements in anatomy. Later, these meetings took place in his welcoming home. Beginning with medical students and later shifting to the faculty, these meetings have continued through the years, for a period with Dr. Meek as leader and then under the stimulus of Dr. Ackerknecht, first professor of the history of medicine. On our library shelves we find 39 leather-bound volumes containing 302 typed essays that have been delivered by 80 authors at these seminar meetings between 1913 and 1956. A considerable number of the papers have been published in appropriate journals.

A developing deafness had long been a handicap to ready communication with Dr. Miller, and he had the hypersensitiveness that so commonly accompanies that infirmity. Even Dr. Miller's warmest admirers admit that he was difficult; many would use stronger terms.[2]

But Dr. Miller did achieve abundantly. When the first edition of *The Lung* appeared, *Time* magazine had this to say of the author: "a chipper, cheerful, deaf little man, almost military in his preciseness and persistence; as high tempered as he is patient, just, exacting, and opinionated." [3] Dr. Miller's bibliography numbers some sixty-six items, most of them on the histology of the lung; each of his favorite early anatomists is also represented. During his long and productive life (1858–1939) he received many cherished honors.

Another early member of the anatomy department and also of the department of zoology was Bennet Mills Allen (Ph.D., University of Chicago, 1903). While at Wisconsin from 1903–13, he worked on the origin of the sex cells and the embryonic development of the ovary and testis in mammals. Later he became professor of zoology at the University of California at Berkeley; there he advanced our knowledge of the influence of glands of internal secretion, especially the thyroid and hypophysis, on body growth.

Dr. Walter Sullivan was born in Ludlow, Maine, July 22, 1885. He received his bachelor's degree at Bates College in 1907, a master's degree at Brown University in 1909, and a doctor of philosophy degree from Brown in 1912. Subsequently he taught anatomy at Western Reserve University, Marquette, and Tufts; he became an assistant professor here in 1920, advancing to professor in 1925. He became Emeritus Professor in 1956.

Walter Sullivan exerted great personal influence on the students of the Medical School. Dr. Frances Hellebrandt writes of her early training here:

There was something unique at Wisconsin. It is difficult to identify that difference and to give it a name. It was not so much what we were taught, but the strength of the men who taught us. The willingness of a Sullivan to meet one night a week for an entire year, so that a physical education student writing a B.S. thesis on the movements of the vertebral column might discourse on this subject.[4]

He was an able teacher with quick sympathy and appreciation. He not only said but did generous things that many will not forget. On several occasions, students who were in trouble were invited to spend a few days in his home, and not infrequently the few days prolonged themselves into a few months. One such student comments, "He showed me how to lead a wholesome life by living it."[5]

Walter Sullivan had broad interests and was well informed in the wide field of anatomical literature. His written contributions were not extensive. The descriptive anatomy of primates and the application of radiology and electromyography to studies of the living human anatomy were probably his most successful contributions. He wrote that the X-ray studies on the living gave a concept of the body as a fluid structure. They made it possible to check conclusions arrived at from observations on the cadaver. "Probably the study on the cerebro-spinal fluid and the one on the movement of the fluid along peripheral nerves were the most exciting."[6] Dr. Sullivan continued throughout his active life to carry on dissections and never lost his skill. It was a pleasure to watch him, as many not in the department were able to do occasionally. He was chary of words and only when he had something to contribute did he break through the characteristic Maine barrier for speech.

On May 20, 1960, Dr. Sullivan received the first Emeritus Faculty Award presented by the University of Wisconsin Alumni Association. These words were inscribed on the hand-illuminated parchment scroll: "In recognition of those rare qualities of mind and heart which made him our distinguished teacher, wise counselor, and warm friend." In presenting the parchment, Dr. Mischa Lustok said, "He has given so much to so many students that there is a little of Walter Sullivan in all of us. We now wish to return something to him."

Theodore Hieronymus Bast was born September 1, 1890, in the farming community of Rockfield, Wisconsin, and died in Madison on January 25, 1959. He received the B.A. degree from Ripon College in 1912 and the Ph.D. in anatomy from the University of Chicago in 1921. He came to the department of anatomy in 1920 and continued his exceptionally active, vigorous life in teaching and research until his death. He always referred to his research work as his "hobby" and considered the teaching of histology to the medical students as his major responsibility. He attacked both his research and his teaching with zeal, leading to high accomplishment in both lines of endeavor. He won the respect of the first-year students who soon discovered beneath his rather abrupt manner a genuine concern for their scholastic and personal welfare.

He published seventy-eight scientific papers, frequently jointly with students and colleagues. In collaboration with Dr. Barry J. Anson of Northwestern University, Bast published a number of papers and an important book, *The Temporal Bone and the Ear*, which gave both men a position of prominence in this field.[7] Accurate large scale models of the minute anatomy of the ear reconstructed from serial histologic sections were one of his splendid contributions to undergraduate and to graduate instruction. The Triological Society at its meeting in Madison, 1965, paid tribute to the work of Dr. Bast for providing a more accurate understanding of the ear, especially for his discovery of the utriculo-endolymphatic valve, known as the valve of Bast. Also mentioned were his well-cultivated hobbies, gardening in the summer, and wood-working and medical history in the winter.[8] Over the years he read more than twenty papers before the Miller medical history seminar; many of these were published. A faculty memorial committee has written, "It can be truly said of Dr. Bast that he was guided by the past, worked in the present, and contributed to the future."

Frederick Denkmar Geist was born in Pittsburgh, Pennsylvania, on September 18, 1895; he took undergraduate work at the University of Pittsburgh and then earned the M.D. degree from Tufts Medical School in 1920. From that date until his retirement in 1961, he worked and taught successfully in the department of anatomy; from 1942 to 1946 he was on leave for military service as a Major in the Medical Corps of the United States Army.

In his earlier years here, his teaching was largely in gross anatomy and in histology. Later he took charge of the course in neuroanatomy and was especially successful in relating the laboratory work to difficult problems in clinical medicine. His competent development of the clinical correlation conference as part of the course in neuroanatomy was a source of satisfaction both to him and to the students. He was didactic and precise both in his dissections and in his discussions. He was a skilled mechanic as well and did exacting work with wood and metal as a hobby.

His chief investigations were in the field of bone repair, nerve degeneration, and the fiber pathways of the nervous system.[9] He was highly regarded both as a teacher and colleague; to our regret, illness forced him to retire in 1961.

Harland W. Mossman, embryologist of note and teacher of distinction, was raised on a farm in western New York state where he became a naturalist at heart, a friend of all living things, fauna or flora. This interest shows up in casual conversations, in his choice of vacation spots, and in more philosophical discussions. After graduation from Allegheny College in Pennsylvania in 1920, he entered the graduate school at Wisconsin in the department of zoology. Here he became deeply interested in embryology and the problems of placental transmission with Professor Michael F. Guyer, who had become immersed in that involved field. He came to the department of anatomy directly from his graduate studies in embryology.

Beginning with his early study on the rabbit placenta and problems of placental transmission,[10] his morphologic and physiologic studies of reproduction have grown steadily both in breadth and depth of understanding with the comparative point of view always prominent. His monograph, "Comparative morphogenesis of the fetal membranes and accessory uterine structures," published in the Carnegie Institution's *Contri-*

butions to Embryology (1937), drew him to the attention of scholars both at home and abroad.[11] This comprehensive survey brought together scattered material of value and formulated concepts that have served as the basis for subsequent investigations throughout the world. His papers and those of his graduate students have covered many aspects of reproduction, both morphological and physiological. A perfectionist himself, he expected similar attention to detail on the part of students. They were frequently more comfortable with the less exacting attitudes of some of the other members of the faculty. The high quality of his scholarship and his fundamental sincerity and interest gradually became manifest to all students, and the mellowing influence of the onrolling years have increased this feeling of deep appreciation.

Although serious in appearance, Mossman has a puckish sense of humor which has given rise to many stories and growing legends. One of the best, the unicorn hoax, arose spontaneously from the gift to him of mule-footed steer hoofs. When two students, who were notorious practical jokers, asked what these were, Mossman replied with perfect seriousness, "Unicorn hoofs." They were manifestly skeptical, but Mossman said, "Would you believe it if you saw the skull?" This was his opportunity; he knew that W. F. Dove of the department of genetics had removed the horn anlage from one side of the head of a steer and grafted the other to the midline. This had resulted in a "unicorn." Mossman borrowed the skull and casually placed it on a bench in his office. The students wandered in, examined and accepted the evidence — as did many of the faculty — before he confessed the hoax. And so we see that the fabulous unicorn did lay his head in the lap of our embryologist.[12]

The textbook in embryology by Hamilton, Boyde, and Mossman has gone through three editions and has now appeared in a Spanish translation.[13] Mossman has been one of the most productive members of the anatomy department and has stimulated many graduate students.

Otto A. Mortensen, professor and chairman of the department of anatomy since 1946, came to this campus as a young man back in 1924, just as our hospital and the four-year Medical School were getting under way. He received both his undergraduate and medical education at the University of Wisconsin (B.S., 1927; M.D., 1929), always with highest honors. As a goodly number of excellent men have done in all the departments, he split the work of the second year of medicine in order to act as student instructor in gross anatomy for two years before going on. After an internship, he returned to Wisconsin and the department in 1930 and has remained here, save for a semester at Johns Hopkins with Dr. Lewis Weed for the investigation of cerebrospinal fluid function. He has served admirably on numerous important committees and since 1951 has borne the additional problems of associate dean. In his warm personal relations with students and in his devotion to teaching he has followed in the footsteps of Dr. Sullivan. The responsibilities of the chairmanship came upon him after World War II when we were passing into the period of the affluent society — increased moneys from federal and other agencies, increased number of students, increased salaries and demands for men in all fields — a period of many and severe adjustments.

Although it is beyond our period, I must mention the splendid new building, the Bardeen Laboratories, dedicated May 17, 1957. These laboratories brought the anatomy department from the attic of Science Hall into close association again with the other departments and gave the anatomy department, with the leadership of Dr. Mortensen, the opportunities for growth that could not otherwise have been achieved.

Despite his many heavy and varied burdens, Dr. Mortensen has carried on his research as well as his teaching and administrative duties. He has made solid contributions to the anatomy of cerebrospinal fluid drainage by way of lymphatic channels and through his electromyographic studies of single neuromotor units.[14]

Meryl M. Miles, as associate professor of anatomy, has an independent teaching laboratory and since 1944 has had full responsibility for all the undergraduate courses in anatomy, including those given for the important paramedical professions — physical medicine, occupational therapy, and physical education. Along with devotion to her teaching, she has carried on X-ray studies on the vertebral column and several types of spinal curvature, including the experimental production of scoliosis in rats and mice. Possibly her more cherished publications are a series of electromyographic recordings during normal voluntary movements.

To form an adequate picture of any department, one should have the panorama of the decades unrolling before him with all those who have contributed, both those in humble positions as well as those with prominent names and achievement. Although one gives thanks for those and to those who have been stimulating, persistent leaders for long periods, always, it seems to me, our students are the important contributors.

Aside from our major objective — the teaching and training of students so that they may meet the requirements for the doctor of medicine degree, the state and national examinations, and, subsequently, the challenges of medical practice — we also have the responsibility, as do all university departments, to train graduate students to explore the limitless frontiers and to serve later on as professional leaders. The anatomy department has been highly successful in furthering all of these aims.

In writing this history, a frustrating limitation imposes itself in that many splendid, productive students have fulfilled only the minor requirements in a given department, such as the anatomy department, and have their major obligation elsewhere. One earnestly wishes to include such students but that would introduce problems that must be avoided.

Following is a list of graduate students who have earned the doctor of philosophy degree with the major in anatomy through 1950.

DOCTOR OF PHILOSOPHY DEGREES FROM THE
DEPARTMENT OF ANATOMY THROUGH 1950

1928	John George Sinclair
1933	Esther Lydia Boyer
1939	Harry Bible Forester
1941	Richard Arnold Groat
	Paul Ellis Nielson
1943	Alice Brownell Eyster
1950	Wilbur George Bingham, Jr.

13 Department of Physiology

For indeed it is one of the lessons of the history of science that each age steps on the shoulders of the ages which have gone before. The value of each age is not its own, but is in part, in large part, a debt to its forerunners. And this age of ours if, like its predecessors, it can boast of something of which it is proud, would, could it read the future, doubtless find also much of which it would be ashamed.

Sir Michael Foster, HISTORY OF PHYSIOLOGY, 1901

From the beginning the department of physiology has been outstanding in our Medical School and highly regarded by other institutions. The faculty has carried a heavy teaching load with zeal and in a spirit of friendly cooperation. Not only have they instructed medical students, but also many fine graduate students to carry the teaching of physiology to other institutions. Students from all other divisions of the University who needed physiology as a part of their training have also been welcomed. The department has fostered investigations in many diverse phases of physiology, from hyperglycemia to energy metabolism in pregnant rabbits, from the effects of certain drugs upon the emptying time of the human stomach to the floating ability of women. The major research interests have commonly been directed to the advance of our knowledge of the heart, cardiac irritability and rhythm.

Dr. Eyster and Dr. Meek were the guiding spirits of our department of physiology; they worked so long and so effectively together that we can hardly think of one without the other. They were, however, markedly different in personality, and I shall try to suggest their differing qualities and some of the distinctive characteristics of their work.

Walter Joseph Meek was born in Dylan, Kansas, on August 15, 1878. He received his bachelor's degree at the University of Kansas in 1902, his master's degree at Penn College, Iowa, in 1907, and the Ph.D. degree at the University of Chicago in 1909. Dr. Meek came to Wisconsin in 1908 to help Erlanger in physiology.

In 1920, Dr. Meek became assistant dean of the Medical School; he effectively presented the needs and problems of our students to Dean Sellery and the College of Letters and Science. His duties included that of advising all premedical students, and he was personally interested in each one of them. Dr. Meek was exceptionally effective in meeting all of the complex demands of his different positions — in teaching, in re-search, in administration, in contacts with other sections of the University and with persons outside the University. His bibliography includes some 109 titles. He worked also with Dr. R. C. Herrin and others in studies on the control of gastrointestinal motility. In collaboration with Dr. Ralph Waters, he worked on problems of anesthesia. With Dr. Seevers in pharmacology, he studied the effects of epinephrin and anesthetic agents, especially cyclopropane on cardiac irritability. He was the only member of that early group — aside from Erlanger and Herbert Gasser, who earned their renown elsewhere — to be elected to the National Academy of Sciences.

A stimulating teacher, both in the laboratory and from the platform, he presented lectures which were lucid and flowed smoothly from one topic to the next. Former President Elvehjem referred to Dr. Meek as "the best classroom teacher under whom I have studied." Dr. Meek retired in 1949, after forty-one years on the faculty of the University of Wisconsin Medical School.

Dr. Meek was a born collector and enjoyed many hobbies, including gardening, bookbinding, and metal working. He gathered an excellent collection of American pewter and made attractive pewter vessels of his own design. He collected stamps avidly.

His published historical studies are delightful reading. One especially enjoyable paper is titled "The Gentle Art of Poisoning." A collection of his historical papers was reprinted for the sixth fall meeting of the American Physiological Society, held in Madison in 1954.[1] In a foreword to that volume, Erwin H. Ackerknecht, formerly our professor of the history of medicine, paid tribute to Dr. Meek, emphasizing the high quality of his historical research.

Walter Meek was a modest, unassuming man, readily approachable both by students and colleagues, and always helpful. He gained the respect and affection of his colleagues, young and old. He died at Fort Myers Beach, Florida, on February 15, 1963, rich in years, accomplishments, and friends. A letter from Dr. Hance Haney provides us with sidelights on his character.

To me Dr. Meek epitomizes Wisconsin. I can think of him only in terms of superlatives. Few men combined the qualities of intelligence, industry, integrity, warmth of personality, loyalty to family, the medical school, friends, and his profession — all of which were so strongly a part of Dr. Meek's makeup. I shall never forget the deep concern he felt for each of his students. One could not work with Dr. Meek without being permanently and importantly influenced by all of these personal characteristics. He loved the yearly physiology picnics and often went to great trouble in arranging for interesting places with beautiful views. The steak fries, softball games, and the great fun of these outings are vividly recalled.[2]

John Augustine English Eyster, the son of a Virginia physician, was born on a farm in Augusta County, Virginia, July 31, 1881, and died in Fort Myers, Florida, March 5, 1960. He received his bachelor's degree from the Maryland Agricultural College in 1899 and his degree in medicine from Johns Hopkins University in 1905. After a year of study at the University of Freiburg, Germany, he returned to the Hopkins, serving with increasing responsibilities in the department of physiology until 1909, when he became professor of pharmacology and toxicology at the University of Virginia. When Erlanger resigned in 1910, Dr. Eyster was named to succeed him here as chairman of the department of physiology.

Dr. Eyster was pre-eminently a scientist and he is the only one of that early group to whom I can apply the word "brilliant." He was able to quickly absorb and later recall in detail whatever he read. He was, however, a poor administrator, ignoring essential details, and soon gave over the chairmanship of the department to Dr. Meek, who handled such tasks with ease and skill.

He was deeply concerned with the effectiveness of his lectures and hoped that they would reach the students. Such was commonly not the case, save for the best students. He did not speak forcibly and he paced back and forth as he spoke, so that his lectures were difficult to follow; he tried to include many recent observations along with the accepted facts.[3]

With Dr. Meek, he produced a long series of significant studies of the conduction mechanism of the heart and the disturbances thereof. The first paper from the collaboration of Eyster and Meek in cardiovascular research was published in 1912 and the last some thirty years later. Most of these studies were concerned with cardiac irritability, the origin and conduction of the cardiac impulse, or bioelectric phenomena in the heart. It is of historical interest that the first article in the first issue of *Physiological Reviews*, 1921, is one by Eyster and Meek, "The origin and conduction of the heart beat."

Eyster's electrocardiography led him to study the injury potentials of the heart. Micro-electrodes have replaced his indirect approach, but his work in this area was a valuable contribution. His studies on myocardial hypertrophy following injury were fundamental. He found that constriction of the thoracic aorta in dogs led to hypertrophy of the left ventricle only after histologic degenerative changes had appeared in the myocardium. His bibliography includes some ninety titles. Among these is an excellent monograph on the clinical aspects of venous pressure.[4]

Following his retirement to Florida, he was plagued by disabling illnesses, but found new outlets for his intellectual curiosity. Astronomy became a preoccupation. He acquired two telescopes, and spent much time getting them in focus. He loved gadgets; possibly he was more interested in making them work than in what he found therewith.

A story from his early days at the University of Virginia suggests his stubborn qualities. When he went there from Hopkins as a young professor of pharmacology he found that the usual schedule of classes was from 9:00 A.M. to 2:30 P.M., at which hour everyone went home to a big dinner and then had the afternoon free for amusements, siestas, or study. Eyster announced that the hours would thereafter be from 8:00 A.M. to 12:00 and 1:30 to 4:30 P.M. In hearing of this disruption of leisurely customs and proper dinners, the boardinghouse keepers revolted. But Eyster stuck stubbornly to the more strenuous Hopkins hours, and even the cooks had to give in.

Courage, obstinacy, and, withal, gentleness and a certain shyness were among his attributes. Even in family troubles, he showed self-control — no outbursts. He hated gossip of any kind. Whatever the occasion, English was always the Virginia gentleman. Especially where the ladies were concerned English was unfailingly courteous. He would spring up to carry a typewriter upstairs, to remove overshoes on a stormy day, or merely to provide a light for a cigarette. He was a true student and scholar all of his life. One of his closest associates wrote, "He had a share of genius and much of the stuff of which a good life is made."

One of Dr. Eyster's intimate younger associates, Dr. Quill Murphy, said he just couldn't think of an appropriate anecdote; then as we walked along together, he said, "He was just the nicest man I ever knew. He just couldn't say or do an unkind thing to anybody." What finer personal tribute could one obtain?

Dr. Eyster deeply disliked the long Wisconsin winters; to this Virginian, they were a hardship. But he loved the land and everything about it, whether in the hunting area of his beloved Shenandoah Valley or on his large farm near Mazomanie, Wisconsin, where he delighted in entertaining his friends. Those who joined him in roaming the hills with hunting dogs, shooting quail in season, were especially welcome guests. He was an enthusiastic and capable gun handler. He loaded his own shells and at one time had ten or fifteen different types of guns. The farm and its many cattle were merely a means to a more important end — hunting and reminiscing with friends.

A comparison of the modes of approach of Eyster and Meek to their experimental problems will interest their students and friends. Dr. Meek loved his teaching and he was deeply interested in each student and his possible development. His position as the one chiefly responsible for admission of students to the Medical School gave him an unusual opportunity to know and to select excellent men as assistants. The lists of younger men in the department through the years and their subsequent growth proves the high quality of his judgment. After choosing the man, Meek sought for the appropriate problem for that man.

Dr. Eyster's approach was quite different; the problem at hand was paramount in his mind. He was interested in ideas rather than men. He was primarily searching for information and the best means of attaining it, as for example when he employed three physicists in the series of experiments which involved mapping the electrical fields surrounding the heart. His methods seem to have been more direct. His major students emphasize the brilliance of his mind. Meek and Eyster trained many fine graduate students who went on to highly successful careers and who retained a warm affection for their former teachers and friends.[5]

Percy M. Dawson was born in Montreal, Canada, on May 19, 1873. He studied at McGill University for several years, but withdrew because of illness and later obtained both his bachelor's degree (1894) and medical degree (1898) from Johns Hopkins University. He remained at Hopkins, advancing in the department of physiology until 1909 when he resigned from his position as associate professor to strike out into a very different field. He studied at Harvard Divinity School for a year and then served for two years as a Unitarian clergyman in Ann Arbor, Michigan. Again, physiology took first place, and he taught in that department from 1913 through 1930, with special responsibility for students majoring in physical education. This became the important field of his teaching and research, his students acting as enthusiastic experimental subjects and junior colleagues. He devised stationary bicycles equipped to record amounts of energy expended and the effects on heart rate, blood pressure, and other bodily functions. He continued such quantitative studies on himself for decades, more recently aided by colleagues at Stanford University. They report, "While there is a decrease of his working capacity during these fifty years, Dr. Dawson's exercise ability at age 91 is comparable to that of a healthy man of 60." [6]

Dawson relished the unconventional. At seminars he would bring out a bag of his socks to darn with three heavy strands of yarn, not necessarily of the same color. A dishevelled appearance was in keeping with his indifference to accepted modes. During the milder months, he ate his lunch of cabbage soup on the wide granite windowsill on the south side of the first floor of Science Hall.

He was ardent in his devotion to exercise and also to a liberal philosophy of life. He was a pacifist, a socialist, and an enthusiastic supporter of many lost causes, including markedly simplified spelling. This last conviction led him into difficulty. From 1930 through 1933, Dr. Dawson obtained leave of absence to write a book, *The Physiology of Physical Education.*[7] Competent reviewers considered the work scientifically excellent, but Percy's insistence that it be published in extreme simplified spelling made it difficult to read and hindered its adoption as a text.

Dawson had a highly retentive, correlating mind, read broadly, and had great charm as a conversationalist. He always loved tramping, whether around Lake Mendota or in the mountains; his colleagues in California report that he and an octogenarian friend still walk about six

miles every Tuesday. He is now working intensively on a detailed autobiography.

Dr. Raymond Clyde Herrin was born in Castleton, Indiana, July 9,
1900; the major part of his student days and his active professional life
have been spent here at the University of Wisconsin. He earned his B.S.
(1922), M.S. (1925), and Ph.D. (1928) degrees here and his M.D.
degree at the University of Chicago in 1933. From 1925 when he became a vigorous part-time assistant in the department of physiology to
the present, he has had a busy and successful career. He earned the
title of professor in 1946. Teaching and research have gone hand in hand
in Herrin's life, and he has always carried his full share of the necessary
smaller tasks of the department. His investigations have covered many
phases of physiology; his special interests have included the role of iron
in nutrition and the emptying time of the stomach under various drug
and diet conditions. His favorite contribution is the work he did with Dr.
Meek published in 1933, "Distention as a factor in intestinal obstruction." Later, he studied the trophic effects of dietary materials such as
protein, amino acids and their related metabolites, and vitamin A upon
renal clearances.[8] Over the years he has presented many valuable papers
in the history of physiology at the Miller history seminar.

Dr. Frances A. Hellebrandt received most of her academic and early
professional training here at Wisconsin with B.S. and M.D. degrees in
1928 and 1929. After Dr. Dawson's retirement in 1930, Dr. Hellebrandt
assumed responsibility for the teaching of physiology to the women students majoring in physical education. She continued to develop an active
productive group.
From 1944 to 1951 she was director of the Baruch Center of Physical
Medicine at the Medical College of Virginia in Richmond and from 1951
to 1955 was head of the department of physical medicine and rehabilitation at the University of Illinois. She tried to retire from professional
life in 1955, but resumed her work here at Wisconsin in 1957. She remained with us until 1964, when she apparently succeeded in retiring.
She continues to devote much time to her violin, which sings beautifully.
Over 150 papers have come from her efforts and those of her associates. They fall into several categories indicating the wide range of her

interests — the physiology of exercise, studies on posture, physical medicine and rehabilitation, and the physiology of motor learning. Her favorite paper, and one highly regarded by her colleagues, is "Methods of evoking the tonic neck reflexes in man," written with Maja Schade and Marie L. Carns.[9]

In 1948, a generous gift from the Wisconsin Alumni Research Foundation gave the Medical School the privilege of naming a man to hold the Charles Sumner Slichter Research Professorship. The man chosen was Clinton N. Woolsey, M.D., who was at that time associate professor of physiology at Johns Hopkins. He has made valuable contributions to our understanding of localization of function in the central nervous system. Dr. Woolsey has been a rare asset not only in the development of neurophysiology but also in tying the Medical School more closely to other divisions of the University. The story of the growth and development of his research unit must be left to future historians.

After the retirement of Dr. Meek (1949) and Dr. Eyster (1952), Dean Middleton and the faculty were especially happy to welcome back one of Meek's former assistants, Dr. William B. Youmans. After undergraduate training at Vanderbilt University and Western Kentucky State College, Youmans came to Wisconsin in 1935 as a WARF fellow and received his Ph.D. degree here in 1938. He received the M.D. degree in 1944 from the University of Oregon. He served on the faculty of that institution from 1938 to 1952 when he was called back to Wisconsin. Although this date is beyond our time limit, we think it desirable in this instance to change our glasses momentarily to see a little farther. Dr. Youmans has happily bridged the decades and is continuing with his associates to maintain a department devoted both to teaching and to research. Among Youmans' many important studies is his monograph *Nervous and Neurohumeral Regulation of Intestinal Motility.*[10]

Quillian Rufus Murphy, Jr., who earned the Ph.D. degree at Wisconsin in 1946 and the M.D. degree in 1948, has continued in the physiology department to aid in carrying on the excellent traditions of teaching and research so well established by Eyster and Meek. His research has included detailed studies in cardiac arrhythmias and also in the autonomic nervous system.

But new blood and genes from other sources are also necessary to meet changing conditions. These have been introduced from California in the person of William Ellis Stone (B.S., 1933, California Institute of Technology; Ph.D. in physiological chemistry, 1939, University of Minnesota). He came to the department in 1947 just early enough for us to be able to mention his fine continuing studies on the chemical physiology of the brain.

Eleanor M. Larsen (A.B., Oberlin, 1924) came into the department of physiology at the beginning of World War II after several years of teaching. Like others during that difficult period, she worked double time without vacations. She earned the Ph.D. degree at Wisconsin in 1948. She has taught physiology not only to the women students majoring in physical education, but also to those studying physical therapy. Her favorite papers are "The fatigue of standing," and "The menstrual cycle length and variability of young adult women."[11]

The department of physiology has been especially productive in training advanced students, in providing minor opportunities for those with major obligations in other departments, and in the awarding of doctor of philosophy degrees to its own graduate students. Between the years 1923 and 1950, thirty such degrees were awarded to men and women who have gone into university circles and into industry with high success.

DOCTOR OF PHILOSOPHY DEGREES FROM THE
DEPARTMENT OF PHYSIOLOGY THROUGH 1950

1923	Ko-Kuei Chen
	Chauncey Depew Leake
	Ethel Ronzoni
1924	Paul Chesley Hodges
1927	Frederick Earl Emery
	Forrest Draper McCrea
	John Allen Wilson
1930	Steven John Martin
1934	Hance Francis Haney
1936	Thomas Cecil Sherwood
1938	William Barton Youmans

1939	Henry Dumke Lauson
	Frank Maresh
	Oswald Sidney Orth
1940	Karl Henry Beyer, Jr.
	Ruth Elizabeth Brogdon
	Carl George Heller
1941	Charles Robert Allen
	Harold Goldberg
	Emily Johnson Heller
	Clarence Alfred Maaske
	Jacob William Stutzman
1943	Kenneth Patrick DuBois
1944	James Arthur Bain
1946	Quillian Rufus Murphy
1948	Eleanor Marie Larsen
1949	Wilbur Maxwell Benson
	James Melford Price
	Maryloo Spooner
1950	Gerald Conrad Mueller

14 Department of Pharmacology and Toxicology

One of the first duties of the physician is to educate the masses not to take medicine.

Man has an inborn craving for medicine. Heroic doses for several generations has given his tissues a thirst for drugs. The desire to take medicine is one feature which distinguishes man, the animal, from his fellow creatures.

Imperative drugging — the ordering of medicine in any and every malady — is no longer regarded as the chief function of the doctor.

Remember how much you do not know. Do not pour strange medicines into your patients.

William Osler

In seeking a competent pharmacologist to be head of a productive department in that field, Bardeen went back to his friends at Johns Hopkins. There he found Arthur Solomon Loevenhart, whom Dr. Bunting delighted in referring to as the "Three Kings." Dr. Loevenhart had received the B.S. degree at the University of Kentucky in 1898 and the M.D. degree at Johns Hopkins University in 1903, where at that time he was an assistant in pharmacology and physiological chemistry. Dr. Loevenhart was born in Lexington, Kentucky, December 29, 1878, and died April 20, 1929, at the age of fifty-one, his untimely death depriving us of many happy productive years with him.

While an undergraduate, Loevenhart published a joint paper with his favorite chemistry professor, J. H. Kastle, on the oxidation of formic aldehyde by hydrogen peroxide and the following year an important communication on the reversibility of enzyme action.[1] Biological oxida-

95

tion became one of the fields of penetrating experimentation throughout his life.

At Hopkins he came under the influence of Dr. John J. Abel, professor of pharmacology, and assisted in the experimental work of the department, thus early choosing his future path. After graduation he remained in the department with increasing achievement until he came to Wisconsin as professor of pharmacology and toxicology in 1908. Dr. Loevenhart's quarters, along with those of Erlanger and Bradley, were for several years in the cramped attic of the old Chemical Engineering building. His generous enthusiasm and ready wit were a life-giving stimulus to the early attic Medical School.

Loevenhart's work at Wisconsin centered around the mechanism of biological oxidation, particularly the stimulation of the medullary centers of respiration: "He observed that substances which reduce oxidation, cause, like anoxemia, a stimulation of the center, provided the center is initially irritable and the change takes place with sufficient velocity. On the other hand, substances containing active oxygen, like sodium iodoxybenzoate, depress the center. He was therefore much impressed with the role played by oxidation in the control of respiration." [2] On these and other observations he elaborated a theory of fundamental importance largely substantiated in further experiments. These gave a basis for later dramatic studies with Dr. William Lorenz when they investigated cerebral stimulation in shock, dementia praecox, and similar states.

During the agonies of World War I and the national terror caused by the unexpected gas attack, Dr. Loevenhart was called to Washington to head the division of pharmacology and toxicology of the Chemical Warfare Service. Arthur established night and day shifts on toxicity testing and the gassing chambers, with the aid of many of his former students. With his customary drive, he gave rapid and efficient handling to the necessarily complex studies, involving also adequate protection of his men.

Among many investigations in the Chemical Warfare Service, studies were made on organic arsenic compounds, some of them never before synthesized.[3] After the war and his return to Wisconsin, Loevenhart continued experimental work on these compounds and their usefulness in treating venereal disease. He and his co-workers collaborated with many different institutions. The clinical facilities of the Wisconsin Psychiatric Institute, the chemical laboratories of Northwestern University and the

Rockefeller Institute for Medical Research, and research funds and other aid from the Interdepartmental Social Hygiene Board of the government, from the private Public Health Institute of Chicago, and Parke, Davis Company were essential. Important aid came also from Drs. Bunting and Clark from the department of pathology.

In the study of arsenical drugs, different species of trypanoscmes were used for screening purposes; experimental syphilitic rabbits served as the test animal. In the long study they discovered the value of tryparsamide in the treatment of neurosyphilis. In a number of compounds studied, Loevenhart traced a relation between structural formulae and spirocheticidal action. These findings led him to propose extension of the work to the founding of a therapeutic institute devoted to finding better methods of treating the sick. Unfortunately, he did not live to make this dream a reality.

Considerable success in treating experimental trypanosomiasis with tryparsamide led to the sending cf one of the collaborators, Dr. W. K. Stratman-Thomas, to try this drug in combating African trypanosomiasis caused by two species of trypanosomes and spread by tsetse flies. This attempt was unsuccessful; as is true in the use of other arsenicals, primary optic atrophy became a serious problem. This effort does, however, show the far-reaching interests of the department.

Shortly after the end of World War I, a long series of experiments on syphilis was undertaken in collaboration with Dr. W. L. Lorenz of the Psychiatric Institute and a changing group of associates. Syphilis was produced in rabbits by Dr. P. F. Clark using the highly invasive strain of *Treponema pallidum* obtained from Dr. H. J. Nichols. These studies were carried on for a year or more in the long bacteriology attic laboratory under the skylights originally constructed to form a greenhouse for the botany department. Later, Stratman-Thomas, Albert Young, and George Wakerlin became the important collaborators; the animals and the team were moved higher up in the great central tower of Science Hall with the responsibilities entirely in the pharmacology department.

Dr. Loevenhart and his associates were exceedingly productive. A spirit of familiar cooperative excitement prevailed, and papers both with and without his name streamed forth, about 130 in all. He edited them meticulously before sending them to journals for publication. Both his first and last published papers were on oxidation, as was his summary lecture in 1915 for the Harvey Society.[4]

Dr. Loevenhart was more effective in dealing with small groups of students and in the laboratory than in lectures. However, his lecture on patent medicine and quackery was a gem that he enjoyed giving annually to the medical students or occasionally to lay groups. It gave him opportunities to tell of the times he had come off victorious in tilts with blustering attorneys in medico-legal cases.

He was a witty story teller; he could squeeze humor out of any situation. Ordinarily he never repeated himself, but there were a few stories, like the one on the Wine of Cardui case, which we required him to repeat again and again. The manufacturers of this "tonic" had made such extravagant claims that finally the American Medical Association brought suit against them with Dr. Loevenhart as the expert witness. In his study of the tonic, aside from some chemical and small animal tests, Dr. Loevenhart had consumed a considerable portion of the "medicine," and could assert that it had the intoxicating effect of ethyl alcohol. As the case developed, the opposing attorney brought up the usual question of who was the best authority — certain textbooks from which he read extracts or the witness. Dr. Loevenhart said quite simply, "I am," whereupon the attorney exploded. After the explosion had subsided somewhat, Dr. Loevenhart turned to the judge and said, "But your honor, I am under oath."

In reminiscing about Dr. Loevenhart, Dr. Bunting has written:

As a companion, Arthur Loevenhart was a joy. His remarkable memory made him a mine of anecdote and story, and his truly marvelous gift for embellishment made him a raconteur without a peer in my acquaintance. No social gathering, with him present, could be dull. If there was humor in any situation, he could extract it. I well remember the equanimity, nay effervescence, with which he met the vagaries of a senile recalcitrant Ford, on the return from a murder trial at which we were both witnesses. Smoke coming up through the floor boards showed us something was wrong, and it proved to be a fire at the outlet of the gas tank on which we had been sitting. That extinguished and repaired, we drove on through the rain until a few miles further we stopped dead in the middle of a mud puddle. After wiping mud and water off a few battery connections, we again got under way; while still several miles from Madison, we found, as darkness fell, that the head lights were short-circuited or blown out, and we had to creep into town lightless and so home by back streets to avoid traffic cops. All, to him a perfect lark.

In court, he was an admirable witness, accurate, lucid, imperturbable, partisan only of what appeared to him the truth. No pettifogging attorney could best him on cross examination. Though he did not treat the situation with levity, he could not resist replying on one occasion when a badgering attorney had insisted that the main function of the stomach was one of mastication: "No, Mr. ———, all the stomach teeth you have are in your mouth." [5]

Arthur Loevenhart's capacity for making friends, his loyalty to those friends, and their affection for him stir the emotions deeply. "A merry heart doeth good like a medicine."

In 1923, the office of state toxicologist was established by an act of the state legislature. Before this time, cases of suspected criminal poisoning often were not investigated because of the inability of the county to obtain a trained and competent toxicologist. At this juncture, Dr. Loevenhart, whose interests in medico-legal toxicology had always been active, seized the opportunity, chose a competent man, Clarence W. Muehlberger, as assistant professor of toxicology (Ph.D., Wisconsin, 1923) and succeeded in getting him appointed also as state toxicologist, a happy example of cooperative state and University service. Muehlberger's investigations included improved chemical tests for alcoholic intoxication and the toxicity of selenium and tellurium. In 1930, when Muehlberger found greater opportunities in Chicago, Dr. Robert P. Herwick (Ph.D., Wisconsin, 1930; M.D., Chicago, 1936) accepted the attractive dual appointment. His studies while here were primarily on the barbiturates. Because of the severe economic depression, the appropriation for the state toxicologist was eliminated in 1933, and Herwick also found greater opportunities in the larger population center of Chicago.

Since that time, the necessary medico-legal studies of chemical nature have been handled on a private fee basis. Here in the University, from 1933 throughout our period and beyond, Dr. Frank Kozelka (Ph.D., Wisconsin, 1933) has been appointed in several departments and has been chiefly responsible for instruction in toxicology throughout the later years of our period. He has also been available for medico-legal cases as a consultant. Dr. Kozelka has been especially skillful in developing micro methods for toxicological and clinical purposes. His studies in anticonvulsants are also considered significant. His present position is that of professor of medicine.

After Dr. Loevenhart's death in 1929, Dr. Arthur Tatum, who had come here from the University of Chicago the year before, became professor and chairman of the department. He had been an instructor here in pharmacology from 1911 to 1913. In Chicago he had been working chiefly on drug addictions, but the laboratory here and its personnel were so well set up for the further study of the chemotherapy of experimental syphilis and trypanosomiasis that he decided to continue this work, especially with arsenicals.

Shortly thereafter, by using the "therapeutic index," instead of absolute toxicity, Tatum and Cooper found that Ehrlich and Hata (1910) had discarded arsenoxide (Mapharsen) too hastily as being too toxic for use in man. Tatum showed that this drug, a very effective spirochetal agent, had a greater margin of safety than the earlier workers had realized.[6] Mapharsen then became the drug of choice in treating several stages of syphilis until it was superseded by penicillin. As Tatum put it, "The moulds have put me out of business."

He then turned his attention to another devastating world disease, malaria, using bird malaria in canaries as the laboratory model — a happy musical change from monkeys. His point of attack was the latent state of the disease, so difficult to understand and so important in malaria as well as in other infectious diseases.[7] The prophylactic use of barbiturates was another of his important fields; he continued his interest in drug addiction, as did his younger associate, Dr. M. H. Seevers.

Later studies of Clausen, Longley, and Tatum showed the significant coaction of bismuth with a variety of arsenical compounds in the treatment of experimental syphilis. They produced primary optic atrophy by the administration of organic arsenical compounds to monkeys, and Longley and Clausen were the first to cultivate trypanosomes in the developing chick embryo.[8]

Dr. Tatum was born on a farm in Iowa and throughout his life, both in practice and precept, followed the simple life, disliking ostentation and social formality. He had a varied professional career teaching in several institutions, earning the Ph.D. degree from the University of Chicago in 1913 and the M.D. degree from Rush Medical College.

Dr. Tatum's hobbies included billiards, played either at home or at the University Club, and gardening, especially the successful hybridizing of African violets. He enjoyed a degree of fluency in Spanish that he continued to employ personally and professionally. In discussing professional life, he maintained that no amount of time spent hurrying around in the laboratory could compensate for time spent sitting with one's feet on the desk. He carried this out in practice. He greatly enjoyed wandering into other laboratories and asking what he called "foolish questions" that made us forget the things we thought at the moment were important and consider broader enigmas. We too enjoyed these interruptions.

He was frugal in his personal as well as in his laboratory affairs. In his lectures to medical students he attempted to reduce the complexities of pharmacology to a few basic principles. Although his remarks could at times be caustic, one of his closest associates for years states, "I cannot remember Tatum raising his voice in anger." [9] He died on November 11, 1955, rich in merited honors. As Shideman has written, "Tatum's contribution to science through both his own work and that of his many students will be a lasting one." [10]

Even though for spatial reasons families cannot be included in this brief history, we must include Nobel Prize laureates. A son, Edward L. Tatum, was awarded that prize in 1958 together with George Beadle and Joshua Lederberg for studies in organization of genetic material in bacteria.

Dr. Maurice H. Seevers was a student of Dr. Tatum's at the University of Chicago, earned both the Ph.D. and M.D. degrees there, and came to Wisconsin in pharmacology with Tatum in 1929. He continued his productive career of teaching and investigations here until 1942, when he accepted the position of professor and chairman of pharmacology at the University of Michigan. Dr. Seevers devoted years to the study of addiction to morphine and other drugs both in dogs and in monkeys. His addicts were always delighted to receive his visits! With Dr. R. M. Waters, he studied the pharmacology of anesthetic gases, especially cyclopropane. Among other investigations, the barbiturates came in for their fair share of experiment.

Dr. Seevers was such a vivid and vocal person that he was enjoyed both by faculty and by students. We deeply regretted his departure to Michigan. His bibliography of over 160 titles is astounding both for the breadth of coverage and also for the penetrating character of his studies.

When Dr. Seevers left Wisconsin for the University of Michigan in 1942, Dr. O. S. Orth, who had been on the staff of our department of physiology since 1936, joined the department of pharmacology, where he worked successfully for many years. Always, however, one of his major concerns was in the problems of anesthesia, and a part of his appointment was in the subdepartment of surgery, anesthesiology. When Dr. Waters retired in 1948–49, Orth went over to the department of anesthesiology as its head. He became a strong leader of that department, continuing until his premature death in 1964. We shall consider his life and work in the chapter on anesthesiology.

Dr. Frederick Earl Shideman came to Wisconsin as a WARF research assistant in pharmacology in 1936 after receiving his B.A. degree from Albion College, Michigan. He earned his Ph.D. degree here in 1941 with Dr. Seevers and subsequently followed Seevers to Michigan where he received the M.D. degree in 1946. His experimental work during this period was largely on morphine and its derivatives. Dr. Shideman returned to Madison as professor of pharmacology in 1952, four years after the end of our historical survey period.

Chauncey Depew Leake, a striking, outgoing young man, a graduate of Princeton and a sergeant in a World War I machine gun company, was ordered in August, 1917, to report to Major English Eyster in Madison. Dr. Eyster, head of a unit of the Chemical Warfare Service, was charged with investigating several of the toxic gases with which the Germans had dumbfounded the Allies, and the young sergeant knew some chemistry. "Sarge" proved himself capable not only in running gas chambers, but also as a diplomat when it was necessary to take over functions from a young lieutenant who knew neither chemistry nor maneuvers.

Leake liked it so well here in Madison that he stayed on in the departments of physiology and pharmacology in positions of increasing success for more than a decade. He earned one of the first Ph.D. degrees in physiology in 1923 and rose into professorial positions with Dr. Loevenhart in the department of pharmacology. His exuberant manner, his excellent teaching, and most importantly, his penetrating studies into acidosis of ether anesthesia and the blood reactions in ethylene and nitrous oxide anesthesia induced Dr. Ralph Waters to come here in charge of anesthesia in the Wisconsin General Hospital and to study some of the underlying problems in this field. To our regret, in 1928, the University of California took Chauncey away from us to build up the pharmacology department at the Medical Center in San Francisco.

His expanding career took him to the University of Texas, then to Ohio State Medical School, and then back to California where he continues to function admirably both in pharmacology and in the history of medicine. But if there are international meetings in the history of medicine or the history of science (he has been president of each of our national societies in those fields) you will probably find him not in San Francisco, but wherever those meetings are being held, quite at home in any country. Dr. Leake's scientific contributions have been in many areas of pharmacology, especially narcotics, anesthesia, and the mechanism of drug action. In the history of medicine, he has also contributed widely, from a paper on Valerius Cordus and the discovery of ether to such books as *The Old Egyptian Medical Papyri* and *Yellow Fever in Galveston, Republic of Texas, 1839.*[11]

One of our splendid early assistants now practicing in Seattle calls Chauncey a "veritable intellectual dynamo," a characterization in which we can agree. We are happy that because of his early days here, we can claim a part of Chauncey Leake and his successes.

Too many younger persons cooperated in many of the departmental studies to give adequate recognition to each in this necessarily brief account. We can include only those who earned the doctor of philosophy degree in the department during the period under immediate observation.

DOCTOR OF PHILOSOPHY DEGREES IN THE
DEPARTMENT OF PHARMACOLOGY THROUGH 1950

1924	Henry Lenzen Schmitz
	Albert Gayland Young
1926	Warren Kidwell Stratman-Thomas
1930	Robert Port Herwick
1931	John Henry Draize
	Richard Homer Fitch
	Arnold Hamilton Maloney
1935	Carl Curt Pfeiffer
1938	Theodore John Becker
	Phyllis Magdalene Nelson
	Harold Willard Werner
1939	Robert Tulloch Stormont
1940	Bruce Jack Longley
1941	Frederick Earl Shideman
	Howard James Tatum

1942   Harold James Byrne
        Norman Martin Clausen
        Charles Henry Hine
1943   James Humphrey Barbour
1944   John Edmund Gajewski
1947   Etta Mae MacDonald
1950   John Edward Steinhaus
        Robert Truman Capps

15   Department of Pathology

Bone, cartilage and connective tissue consist in the same
way *of cells and intercellular substance. The cells appear
round, oval, lentiform, tailed, branched and forming
anastomoses; the intercellular substance appears hyalin,
granular, bandy and fibrillated. The former resist cooking,
the latter becomes first homogenized, then dissolved.*
Rudolf Virchow, CELLULAR PATHOLOGY, 1863

In the second year of the medical course, students come
face to face with the end results of disease at the autopsy table. There
the damaged organs are examined grossly and later microscopically; attempts are made to correlate the symptoms and signs described by patient and physician with the findings as seen by the pathologist. Although
the department of pathology was instituted with the appointment of Dr.
Bunting in 1908, fresh autopsy material was meager until the Wisconsin
General Hospital was opened in 1924. Until 1935 medical bacteriology
was also a part of the department of pathology; then it was renamed
medical microbiology and given departmental status. Because of the lack
of post-mortem opportunities, few of the younger members of the pathology department stayed for any considerable time until after the Wisconsin General Hospital was completed. With deep personal regret, we must
omit them all for lack of space.

Dr. Charles Henry Bunting (1875–1961), a naturalist and scholar
at heart, a physician and pathologist by profession, was our first professor of pathology, a position he held for thirty-seven years. After
receiving a B.S. degree at the University of Wisconsin in 1896, always
at the top of his class, he took a year's fellowship with Professor E. A.

Birge as mentor before going on to obtain the M.D. degree in 1901 at the Johns Hopkins Medical School. He studied under the wise leadership of "Popsy" Welch (Dr. W. H. Welch) at the Hopkins for several years, and continued his training in pathology with Dr. Simon Flexner at the University of Pennsylvania. He especially enjoyed this Pennsylvania period with his gay associates — Dr. John Lawrence Yates, of sharp, spicy speech, Dr. Richard Pearce, and Flexner's little Japanese shadow, Dr. Hideyo Noguchi, whom Yates, to Noguchi's great delight, dubbed "The Yellow Peril." Together at the local "pub" they carried on Noguchi's education in English with well-chosen limericks and with the formation of the "Society for the Liberation of Captive Balloons"; Noguchi needed no help from them either in capturing or in liberating balloons!

After two years as professor of pathology at the University of Virginia, Bunting was brought back to Wisconsin by Bardeen in 1908 to join the small group, mostly from Johns Hopkins, who were building up the productive two-year school of medicine. Here he remained with only occasional trips back to Baltimore, or to Maine, where Mrs. Bunting, also a former Hopkins student, had lived and practiced medicine. He always stated that he was never going to get farther away from clinical medicine than pathology would permit.

Dr. Bunting's major scientific interests lay in the diseases of the blood-forming system, especially the lymphoid tissues; of his more than forty publications over half dealt with the hematopoietic tissues and their diseases. With Dr. J. L. Yates of Milwaukee, he worked for many years on Hodgkin's disease, its cytology, blood picture, and possible etiology.[1] Repeatedly they succeeded in isolating diphtheroid organisms from affected glands of the patients. Using these organisms, they observed in their experimental animals changes in the tissues and a blood picture "in perfect agreement with those seen in early Hodgkin's disease." However, they did not succeed in producing the chronic lesions and realized that while their concept of the etiology was attractive, it required proof. As studies have accumulated, they have shown that both the normal and diseased lymph nodes carry a wide variety of micro-organisms, including diphtheroids, but the evidence is insufficient to incriminate any one organism with Hodgkin's disease. Because of Dr. Bunting's sensitive nature, he tended at times to forget that the great Dr. Welch (in hog cholera) and many other competent, distinguished men have made similar errors in judgment.

The care and thought with which Dr. Bunting prepared his lectures resulted in models of clarity: they were rich in historical background and so well organized that students found note-taking easy. With admirable skill he tied clinical findings to tissue and organ damage. He was devoted to teaching. In discussing research with his associate Dr. Gorton Ritchie, he once said, "The people of Wisconsin pay me my salary to teach medical students. If I have time and energy over and above that, I will do research." A very different attitude from the modern one of "publish or perish"! In discussing retirement with Ritchie, he once remarked that retirement would be a great relief to him in two respects, as an escape from "eight o'clock classes and deans." [2]

As part of the regular instruction in pathology, the Junior class was once attending an autopsy with Dr. Bunting as pathologist and Dr. Middleton as clinician. Dr. Middleton as usual had drawn a dividing line on the blackboard. One side read "clinical findings," and the other "autopsy findings." In due course Dr. Bunting opened the heart, examined it, and without looking up said, "There should have been a soft, blowing, systolic murmur heard at the apex and transmitted to the axilla." And then looking up with that quizzical, sophisticated expression that was his alone, he noticed that the clinical findings were blank at this point. He then said, "You know, Bill, they're making stethoscopes with amplifiers these days!" The effect was electric; the class hooted. Dr. Middleton reddened, but without giving an inch, said, "Well, since you're in that mood!" And there followed a series of snappy questions to show who was in charge! [3] From that time on, for that class, Dr. Bunting could do no wrong.

Recalling his University undergraduate contacts, he was especially happy to serve as faculty member of the Wisconsin Athletic Council for many years. In the framework of a devoted family, Dr. Bunting possessed a deep sense of loyalty to his associates and friends. He was not strongly energetic but worked consistently, always taking time for reading not only the immediate journals but broadly in the classics. His microscope bench was a clutter of slides from many sources, but if a question about a given case arose he could always put his hand on the essential slides.

Medical history was one of Bunting's special interests; his scholarly essays read before the Miller history seminar merited publication, but he rarely sent them to journals. During several years he gave a series of delightful lectures in medical history with special emphasis on the old Greek philosophers.

After retirement Dr. and Mrs. Bunting went to New Haven, following their son Henry, a graduate in medicine from Harvard, who was doing excellent work in pathology at Yale. To the regret of all, Henry died in 1954, seven years before his father. He left fine children to carry on. His widow, Mary Ingraham Bunting, is president of Radcliffe College and has served as a member of the Atomic Energy Commission.

Dr. Bunting's last letter to me emphasized his continuing interest in blood. He said that he went to the local hospital at Princeton, New Jersey, frequently, to spend most of his time "playing with blood smears, diagnosing sex, etc." [4] Of all Dr. Bunting's papers, the one he referred to most often was "The fate of the lymphocyte," with John Huston, and later the one that he personally appreciated the most was one written in 1953 with his son, "Acid mucopolysaccharides of the aorta." [5]

Dr. Edgar M. Medlar, who had previously had wide experience, especially in the pathology of tuberculosis, joined Dr. Bunting in 1924. He was born in Ohiova, Nebraska, on March 9, 1887, and died on June 30, 1956. He resigned as professor of pathology in 1927 to continue more intensive studies in tuberculosis as pathologist and director of the Hegeman Memorial Laboratory at Mount McGregor, New York. Medlar's investigations in tuberculosis have been especially wide; they have included study of the disease in man, in cattle, and in experimental animals, many of them unnatural hosts for this disease. In considering the relative importance of allergy and immune phenomena in reinfection, he stresses dosage and the virulence of the particular strain of tubercle bacillus more than do some investigators. In a large series of cases that came to autopsy following sudden and unexpected death, Medlar demonstrated the chronicity of chronic caseous foci; these may persist for years in an unhealed state without significant effect upon the health of the individual. His extensive studies in cattle and other animals showed the effect of posture on the apical localization of progressive tuberculosis.

His extensive bibliography and his monograph, *The Behavior of Pulmonary Tuberculosis Lesions*, are monuments to the intelligent, critical, persistent efforts of this distinguished pathologist.[6] In 1954 he was awarded the Trudeau Medal, the highest honor that can be bestowed by the National Tuberculosis Association.

Dr. Gorton Ritchie, a member of the pathology department during two periods, was born in Oak Park, Illinois, February 15, 1901. After a year at Princeton University, he came to the University of Wisconsin, where he earned the B.A. degree in 1924. He took his first two years of medicine here and completed his clinical years at the University of Pennsylvania, receiving the M.D. degree in 1927. He returned to Wisconsin to join Dr. Bunting in pathology and advanced in the department until 1939 when he went to the Racine Hospitals for more extensive autopsy experience. During the war years, he returned to Wisconsin (1943) to take charge of the pathology department. With the reorganization of the department after World War II, he resigned as professor of pathology to become pathologist of Columbia Hospital in Milwaukee.

One of his favorite papers suggests his major interest in tumor pathology, "Argentaffin tumors of the gastrointestinal tract."[7] His chief concerns tended to follow those of Dr. Bunting — fidelity to teaching and much reading in the classics, both in medicine and in the humanities.

Dr. John McCarter joined Dr. Bunting and the pathology department in 1934. He was born in Duluth, Minnesota, on May 19, 1904, obtained his B.A. degree in 1930 and the M.D. degree in 1932, both from Wisconsin. After an internship at Kansas City General Hospital, McCarter returned to Wisconsin, first being associated for a year in gross anatomy with Dr. Sullivan and subsequently, for almost a decade, in the pathology department with Dr. Bunting. He had a valuable experience in neuropathology, a Rockefeller fellowship at McGill University in 1939–40, and from then began to specialize in that field. He introduced a course in neuropathology for the third-year students and a review conference in gross pathology for the fourth year. He rose in rank to associate professor before leaving in 1943 for a position elsewhere.

One of his favorite papers was "Brain tumors in Wisconsin," published in 1936 with Dr. Mead Burke.[8] He writes, "My chief efforts were in teaching, for which I respected Dr. Bunting, the finest teacher in medicine that I knew." [9]

Dr. Mead Burke was born in Chicago, Illinois, September 17, 1894. He received his B.A. degree at the University of Wisconsin in 1917, took his first two years of medicine here, and then completed his training for the M.D. degree at Rush Medical College, Chicago, in 1928.

After several years in private practice, he served in the department of pathology from 1933 until 1942. Then for two years, he did an important job as chief resident and assistant superintendent of the Wisconsin General Hospital with Dr. Buerki. His detailed study of overcrowding in the hospital with its effect on infections gave a basis for helpful changes.

While in the pathology department he devoted much time to analysis of the departmental statistics on cancer, especially multiple cancer in the individual. His most cherished publication, "Thrombosis — a medical problem," called attention to the importance of this vascular damage not only in surgical but also in medical cases.[10]

In 1944 Dr. Burke left the University for study and experience in allergy; he subsequently returned to Madison and has continued to practice that specialty successfully with his wife, Myra Emery Burke (M.D. Wisconsin, 1927).

At the end of World War II, Dr. D. Murray Angevine was appointed professor and chairman of the department of pathology (October, 1945), leading us into the era of expansion in this department. Dr. Angevine was born in St. John, New Brunswick, October 8, 1905, and had his early college and medical training in Canada (A.B., Mount Allison University, and M.D., McGill University, 1929). Before he came here, he had extensive and varied experience in pathology at Cornell, the University of Pennsylvania, New York Hospital, the DuPont Institute in Wilmington, Delaware, and in the Medical Corps of the Army of the United States during World War II.

He has built up an active teaching and experimentally productive department to which, because of our time limitations, we may give only a slight introduction. Angevine's interests are broad, both in human relations and in pathology. Diseases of connective tissue with special reference to the pathology of the skeletal system have been his continuing interest.[11]

The men now in pathology who derive in part from the earlier period here are Dr. Walter Jaeschke (M.D., Wisconsin, 1934) and Dr. Joseph

Lalich (M.D., Wisconsin, 1937). Jaeschke worked with Dr. Bunting for two years and has long been the highly effective and much appreciated pathologist of the hospital. Lalich did graduate work here with Dr. Eyster, but went on in pathology at Kansas Medical School with Dr. Ralph Major and returned here to join Dr. Angevine after World War II. Dr. Edward Asahiel Birge, Jr. (B.A., Wisconsin, 1932; M.D., Johns Hopkins, 1936), grandson of former President Birge, was in clinical pathology from 1940 through 1947, when he resigned to become director of the laboratories of Milwaukee Hospital.

16 Department of Physiological Chemistry

*Does Science leave no mystery? On the contrary, it
proclaims mystery where others profess knowledge. There
is mystery enough in the universe of sensation and in its
capacity for containing those little corners of consciousness
which project their own products, of order and law and
reason, into an unknown and unknowable world. There is
mystery enough here, only let us clearly distinguish it from
ignorance within the field of possible knowledge. The one
is impenetrable, the other we are daily subduing.*
Karl Pearson, GRAMMAR OF SCIENCE, 1892

In 1878 when R. H. Chittenden went to Germany as a
young student to study the possible applications of chemistry to physiology, biochemistry had no real standing in this country. Gradually the
scene and the emphasis changed, especially in those institutions where the
physiologists had had the opportunity for European study. Now almost
every project seems to demand a detailed knowledge of that field
and the methods. It is obvious that our first professor of physiological
chemistry foresaw some of this change in attitudes.

Harold Cornelius Bradley was born in Oakland, California, November 25, 1878, the son of a professor in the University of California at
Berkeley. Whether by nature or by nurture, Bradley always had to an
exceptional degree the broader interests of the University and the students both in heart and in mind.

From the University of California (B.A., 1900), Bradley crossed
the continent to Yale, where physiological chemistry was becoming a distinct discipline under the guiding hands of R. H. Chittenden, T. B. Os-
borne, and Lafayette B. Mendel. In his investigations, Bradley worked

chiefly with Mendel, and together they published three fine papers on certain underlying factors in digestion and in self-digestion, autolysis. With his Ph.D. degree (1905) he accepted the call of Dr. Erlanger the next year to take charge of physiological chemistry in the projected medical school at Madison. Erlanger states that he was having a difficult time getting organized in the bare attic laboratories and in preparing to give the entire course in physiology, a responsibility that he had not had previously, and that he was delighted to receive Bradley's help.[1] Harold insists that he really did not come into Madison on skis, and since he came in October, I must accept that statement. But he does admit that he soon learned to use them, and I am sure we all think of the skiing Bradleys, the Sierras, the Tuolumne Meadows, and the conservation movement in the same moment.

Dr. Bradley took up his new duties with characteristic enthusiasm. Those were simpler days; there were no automobiles, and medicine in Madison required little apparatus. In reminiscing about these early days, he says:

As soon as I had a laboratory and sufficient equipment to carry on chemical work — with necessary glassware, chemicals, microscopes, balances and the like — Bardeen suggested that I might offer some routine laboratory tests to the city physicians. So I held several meetings with the local doctors and proffered them our help along such lines, if they were desired, as a free service in the aid of diagnosis. Usually such tests would be for sugar or albumin or ketone compounds in the urine, perhaps a microscopic examination of the sediment for red blood cells, pus, and other significant items.

I soon found myself fairly busy and happy to get to know the doctors better, and now and then to sit in as a consultant on the significance of the findings. One day, a fruit jar came in with a urine sample and on the bottom a small handful of dark colored hard objects that looked suspiciously like crushed limestone then being used to surface our city streets. The doctor wanted to know the nature of these "stones" and whether they were of kidney or bladder origin. They were crushed limestone all right, and I never was quite sure whether the doctor was trying out the reliability of our free laboratory service or whether the patient was trying out the doctor.[2]

He tells of another amusing incident brought about by the need for a larger Madison General Hospital. As president of the hospital board, Bardeen asked Bradley to push a membership drive to obtain funds for a sorely needed new wing for the hospital. Under Bradley's initiative the campaign progressed merrily. One device that he had thought pretty clever — the printing of a large red cross across the face of the membership card — caused him no small embarrassment when Bardeen informed him that the red cross was a copyrighted symbol and could not be used. So the illegal cards were recalled, and a new design substituted. The campaign was highly successful despite this minor contretemps. Bradley recalls, "We organized a number of public meetings when Bardeen explained modern hospital uses and needs and urged membership and active interest in securing and equipping the new building. Those meetings did much to provide better understanding also of the Medical School."[3]

Reflecting on his University life in Madison, Bradley writes, "I loved to teach. I loved to do the kind of research I did do. I enjoyed my twenty years or so with the Wisconsin Union and acting as one of the founders of its outing group, the Hoofers." Bradley also served as chairman of the committee that finally achieved the first men's dormitories along the lake and established the excellent system of dormitory fellows. He was active on many committees that studied and contributed to the betterment of student life. He says that his membership on the Athletic Council was a joke because he wanted to abolish intercollegiate athletics and promote participant sports and a program in physical education.[4]

Teaching in the laboratory and in intimate seminar groups were Dr. Bradley's favorite activities. Along with his teaching went investigations in digestion, especially in autolysis. Curti and Carstensen state with due appreciation of Bradley's role in our small beginnings that "to gain recognition for his relatively small department in the shadow of a much stronger and extremely successful biochemistry department in the College of Agriculture was no mean task."[5] But we in the Medical School family hardly realized that; we were all small together.

Chittenden, one of the fathers of physiological chemistry in this country, wrote, "Bradley's work and that of his associates has contributed much to an understanding of the conditions which influence autolytic changes and has thrown light upon the character and extent of the processes involved."[6] His studies have shown the importance of trace elements such as manganese, copper, and zinc, as well as the H-ion concentration on the intracellular proteolytic enzymes involved in the autolysis of tissues both in vertebrates and in invertebrates. His work represented a substantial beginning in our understanding of atrophy as a physiologic and pathologic function.[7] Bradley's important work in the gas warfare service of World War I is presented in Chapter Four.

Almost universally in the histories of medical schools, the faculty families, although manifestly of underlying importance, are thought to be in a different field and are not considered save when they come professionally or directly into the picture. In the Bradley family we have such an instance. In 1916, they were heart-broken, as many other families have been, by the sudden death of their lovely seven-year-old daughter, Mary Cornelia Bradley. They and we were fortunate, however, in that they had family funds to build the Bradley Memorial Hospital for the investigation and treatment of children's diseases as a continuing remembrance. I well remember the occasion, probably early in 1917, before the United States entered World War I, when we followed Bardeen, Bradley, and Evans up the hill to be greeted by President Van Hise and to hear the announcement of the wonderful gift. We were overjoyed to realize that at long last, and despite opposition, the first building was to be constructed for clinical purposes quite beyond infirmary needs of the students. Before it was completed, "the Bradley" was used in 1919 to care for some of the influenza cases in the great 1918–19 pandemic.

Following Bradley's retirement from the Medical School in 1949, he returned to Berkeley and devoted himself effectively to what had previously been his major hobby, the out-of-doors — the mountains, wild life, and conservation. Back in January, 1921, he made the first solo ski trip that we know of across the Sierras. In so-called retirement he now had the time, the courage, and the vital interest to aid in preserving some of this great natural resource for others. It has been a wonderful new career and a fruitful one; he has published papers, held meetings, and entered the political turmoil to preserve some of our vanishing heritage.[8] We are indeed grateful that Harold Bradley came to Madison and that he continues his strong influence in this second career.

Dr. Bradley was the first (1906) and Dr. W. J. Meek the second (1908) appointee to our medical school faculty with the specialized training leading to the doctor of philosophy degree. After years of study by the American Medical Association Council on Medical Education, the chairman, Dr. A. D. Bevan, had emphasized the necessity of improved laboratory training in the underlying sciences commonly taught in the first two years of the medical course. This was further stressed in the pungent, objective reports of Abraham Flexner in 1910 and 1912. Enough graduates in medicine with additional training in the underlying sciences were not available for the increasing demands of medical education, so that appointments without training in clinical medicine became frequent here and throughout the land. These men have done well, some of them rising even to the high honor of the Nobel Prize. It is encouraging to observe, however, that over the period of our history and beyond, an increasing number of such specially trained men have also earned the doctor of medicine degree as an aid to bridging the difficult gap between the preclinical and the clinical types of training.

Dr. Elmer L. Sevringhaus grew up scientifically with Dr. Bradley in the department of physiological chemistry. After completing the work for the M.D. degree at Harvard in 1916, he returned to serve well in this department for six years. He then left the quieter academic field to take on clinical responsibilities in the department of medicine where he carried on successfully for a longer period, about two decades. Because of this longer service his story of achievements will be told in the chapter on the department of medicine.

Dr. Edgar J. Witzemann (1884–1947) joined the department of physiological chemistry in 1927 after spending sixteen years as a research chemist associated with the Sprague Memorial Institute for Medical Research at the University of Chicago and with the Mayo Foundation in Rochester, Minnesota. He received his bachelor's degree at Millikin University in 1907, and at Ohio State University he received the Ph.D. degree in 1912. One of Witzemann's early achievements while at Chicago was the working out of the method for the preparation of large quantities of pure crystalline glyceric aldehyde, which was being considered as a possible sugar substitute for diabetics. Also related to investigations on diabetes, he began a series of studies on the oxidation of fats which he continued at the University of Wisconsin. As an organic chemist, he did valuable work as a civilian with the Chemical Warfare Service during World War I.

His pleasure in teaching was evident to his students, who appreciated his keen thinking, his interest in sharing their problems, and his gentle humor. Dr. Witzemann enjoyed broadening his knowledge of the history of science and contributed regularly to the Miller history seminar. His philosophical approach to science and history is evident in articles such as "The so-called scientific method and its role as a process in democracy," and "Chemistry and evolution." A representative paper dealing with his scientific work on the oxidation of fats, "A unified hypothesis of the reciprocal integration of carbohydrate and fat catabolism," was published in 1942.[9]

Although Dr. Witzemann's activities focused on his teaching, research, and writing, his wide interests and sense of responsibility extended to the community and the country through his support of welfare and social service projects.

Dr. Philip P. Cohen returned to the University of Wisconsin, where he had taken his Ph.D. (1937) and M.D. (1938) degrees, as a research associate in 1941 and became chairman of the department of physiological chemistry in 1948. He had been a research fellow at Sheffield University, England, and an instructor at Yale University (1938–41), a pioneer institution in physiological chemistry in this country. His primary studies here have been in the intermediary metabolism of proteins and amino acids, and with colleagues he has published about 150 papers. Cohen and his associates initiated studies on urea biosynthesis which demonstrated for the first time the nature of the enzymatic steps involved and which led to the discovery and the characterization of the enzymes carbamyl phosphate synthetase (and its cofactor) and ornithine transcarbamylase.[10] They also did pioneering research on biosynthesis of model peptide bond compounds such as hippuric and ornithuric acids. Beyond our period, he continues active leadership in his field and in the Medical School.

Another productive scholar in the department, Dr. Harold Deutsch, received his training in physiological chemistry at the University of Wisconsin, earning the Ph.D. degree in 1944 and remaining with the department thereafter. His major research has been on the separation and physical characterization of serum, egg white, and milk proteins, and on the quantitative immuno-chemistry of a number of these proteins. He has traveled widely for professional purposes, having served as fellow and visiting professor at the Universities of Brazil and São Paulo and at the Nobel Medical Institute in Stockholm, Sweden. Of his important bibliography, only one rather typical paper can be cited — a procedure for the isolation of a new globulin from normal human plasma.[11]

Dr. Edgar S. Gordon was a member of the department from 1937 to 1940, but later transferred to clinical work in the department of medicine. His major activities will be presented with that department.

With the increasing demand for biochemists, many graduate students have been trained in this department. The following have received the doctor of philosophy degree during the period to 1950.

DOCTOR OF PHILOSOPHY DEGREES IN THE DEPARTMENT OF PHYSIOLOGICAL CHEMISTRY THROUGH 1950

1924	Alrick Brynhjolf Hertzman
1926	Merse Starr Nichols
1929	Harry Daniel Baernstein
1932	Marian Esther Stark
1933	Jane Cape
	Leita Davy
1937	Philip Pacy Cohen
1939	Mary Locke Petermann
1940	Rovelle Harper Allen
	Basil Edwin Bailey
	Robert Norman Feinstein
	Irene Elsie Stark
1941	Arthur Edward Heming
1942	Albert Lester Lehninger
1943	Harold Abbott Wooster
1944	Harold F. Deutsch
1945	Walter Carl Schneider
1947	Robert Warren McGilvery
1948	Mika Hayano
1949	Lemar Fred Remmert
	Adolph Abrams
	Harlan Lyle Klug
	Margaret Eleanor Marshall
1950	Sam Sorof
	Erich Hirschberg
	Leslie Robert Wetter

17 Department of Medical Microbiology

*There are many seeds of things that support our life, and
on the other hand, there must be many flying about that
make for disease and death.*
Lucretius, DE RERUM NATURA, BOOK VI

*There exist in the air minute animals too small to be seen,
but which can penetrate into the mouth and nose, and cause
disease.*
Varro, 116–27 B.C.

In 1914, medical bacteriology was transferred from the
College of Letters and Science to the Medical School, and Dr. Paul F.
Clark was brought here from the Rockefeller Institute to take charge of
this field. Medical bacteriology remained a part of the pathology department until 1935 when, under Dean Middleton, it was made a separate
department. In 1946 the name was changed to the more appropriate one
of medical microbiology, with additional support provided to give greater
emphasis to the helminths and other animal parasites.

Paul Clark was born on the rocky coast of Maine, in Portland, on
May 9, 1882.[1] He went to Brown University in 1900 and continued there
for nine years, earning three degrees: bachelor's, master's, and the
doctor of philosophy degree in 1909. While studying at Brown, he was
also, for a year or two, bacteriologist in the Rhode Island Board of Health
laboratory, carrying on some of the bacteriologic aids in the diagnosis
of the common diseases of that period, such as throat cultures for diphtheria, sputum smears for tuberculosis, and the Widal test for typhoid
fever. His chief investigation at Brown was in the diphtheria group of
bacteria.

119

With the opportunity to work with Dr. Simon Flexner, he went to the Rockefeller Institute in 1909 and, save for a semester's leave of absence for work in pathology at Johns Hopkins, he remained at the Institute until he came here in 1914. At the Rockefeller, his investigations were concerned chiefly with experimental poliomyelitis, which had at that time just been reproduced in monkeys.

He has been happy here at Wisconsin, both in his personal associations and in his professional opportunities; he has thoroughly enjoyed his teaching, his contacts with students, and his investigations. His experimental studies have been largely in virus diseases, especially poliomyelitis and some of the virus encephalitides. He came here as associate professor and was advanced in 1918 to full professorship. He greatly appreciated his associations with Dr. Bunting and the other members of the pathology department. Dr. Clark's professional papers with his associates number about fifty-five; he has published three books, *Alice in Virusland, Memorable Days in Medicine,* written with Mrs. Clark, and *Pioneer Microbiologists in America.*[2]

Development of the department was slow, with much teaching. As Osler said, "Undoubtedly the student tries to learn too much, and we teachers try to teach him too much — neither, perhaps, with great success."[3] Clark was conscientious, with long hours at the bench and library. The graduate student seminar was small enough so that it was for years held intimately in his home. As Curti and Carstensen said of Bradley and the physiological chemistry department, the older, larger, and stronger department of bacteriology in the College of Agriculture made it difficult for the younger department of the Medical School to shine. Also, like Bradley, Clark served on many University committees and functions distinct from those of the Medical School. At various times he traveled on three continents; he worked for brief periods in the laboratory of Jules Bordet at the Pasteur Institute in Brussels and at Cambridge University in the laboratory of G. H. F. Nuttall.

Aside from virus diseases, two early papers in other fields may be cited. One that provided the basis for the design of modern drinking fountains showed that bacteria introduced into a vertical bubbler danced there threateningly, but that this minor hazard could be avoided by tilting the column at an angle of about 55° from the vertical.[4] A paper with Mrs. Clark in the early days of bacteriophage describes such an agent isolated from Madison sewage, active against a virulent hemolytic streptococcus. The hopes for a therapeutic agent were dashed when the animals treated with the specific phage died before the controls.[5]

In the field of public hygiene, the catalogues have described the following course:

> In conjunction with the staff of the State Laboratory of Hygiene, the State Board of Health, and the Board of Health of Milwaukee, courses in hygiene are offered by members of the Faculty of the Medical School under the general supervision of Dr. Clark.[6]

A decade later Dr. Stovall was placed in charge of this work. Curti and Carstensen remark, "Yet the specific goal of training public health officers, stated stubbornly in all programs from 1911 to 1937, did not materialize, as prospective candidates preferred special schools in the field which had been endowed elsewhere."[7] Actually little in the way of separate work was ever offered, and few students ever applied.

Frances E. Holford joined the department in 1923 and has continued well beyond our time limit as a valuable member who has advanced through the years in responsibilities and position. She became an associate professor in 1942. She has always had a deep interest in each student and his needs. She earned the Ph.D. degree in the department in 1929 with a thesis on the placental transmission of foreign protein in rabbits. A later study on antibody response to hemoglobin absorbed on aluminum hydroxide was also significant.[8] Her gracious personality and quick correlations have made her a splendid teacher, especially in her favorite course, immunology.

Hobart W. Cromwell came here with an Sc.D. degree from Johns Hopkins School of Hygiene in 1922, was advanced to assistant professor in 1926, and left here for a commercial position in 1929. He was competent and effective both in teaching and in his investigations. His study of quantitative relationships in the precipitin reaction was one of his favorite studies.[9]

Dr. Charles Victor Seastone (B.A., Wisconsin, 1927; M.D., Harvard, 1932) returned to his native state from the Rockefeller Institute at Princeton as an assistant professor in 1939. He was advanced to associate professor in 1942, was on military leave from 1942 to 1945, and returned in 1945 with promotion to professor. He followed Clark as chairman of the department in 1947, in which post he has done an excellent job. Since the subsequent years are beyond our period, further comment will be left largely for later historians. His more important investigations have been with the hemolytic streptococci, group A, and also group C hemolytic streptococci of animal origin.[10] He has always been the devoted artist in his avocations — music, photography, and pottery.

Dr. A. F. Rasmussen, Jr., came here as a graduate student in 1940 and has done splendid work in all capacities. He earned his Ph.D. in this department, and his M.D. in 1944, also from Wisconsin. He continued here with a year's leave for war work, advancing to a professorship in this department and in preventive medicine at a time just beyond our period. His investigations were largely in experimental virus diseases of the central nervous system, especially poliomyelitis. In a long series of relatively unproductive studies on the influence of diet on experimental poliomyelitis and other virus diseases of the central nervous system, carried on with Conrad Elvehjem, Harry Waisman, and others handling the nutritional side, one example must suffice. Thiamine deficient mice showed a lower incidence of infection to Theiler's virus and to Lansing strain poliomyelitis virus than did the animals fed a similar diet with optimum thiamine.[11] To our regret, Dr. Rasmussen left us in 1952; he is now chairman of the department and professor of infectious diseases at the University of California at Los Angeles.

DOCTOR OF PHILOSOPHY DEGREES IN THE DEPARTMENT OF MEDICAL MICROBIOLOGY THROUGH 1950

1929	Frances Elizabeth Holford
1932	Chun Chieh Young
1935	Arthur Wain Frisch
1937	William Samuel Preston
1939	Harold Victor Ellingson
	Gordon Worley
1941	Aaron Frederick Rasmussen, Jr.
1943	Edward Harold Kass
1947	Paul Donaldson
	Doralea Harmon
	Edna Kearney

1947	Joaquin Munoz
1949	William Arthur Pierce, Jr.
	Morris Dumoff
1950	Wayburn Stewart Jeter
	William Lewis Pond

18   Wisconsin Psychiatric Institute, Department of Neuropsychiatry

The longer I live the more do human beings appear to be fascinating and full of interest. . . .

Foolish and clever, mean and almost saintly, diversely unhappy — they are all dear to my heart; it seems to me that I do not properly understand them and my soul is filled with an inextinguishable interest in them. Many of them whom I knew are dead. I am afraid that except me there is no one who will tell their story as I would like to do and dare not; it will seem as though such men had never existed on earth at all. . . .

The people I am most fond of are those who are not quite achieved; who are not very wise, a little mad, "possessed." "The people of a sound mind" have little interest for me. The achieved man, the one perfect like an umbrella, does not appeal to me. I am called and doomed, you see, to describe — and what could I say of an umbrella but that it is of no worth on a sunny day?

A man slightly possessed is not only more agreeable to me; he is altogether more plausible, more in harmony with the general tune of life, a phenomenon unfathomed yet, and fantastic, which makes it at the same time so confoundedly interesting.

Maxim Gorki

Back in 1910 a brawny young man of twenty-eight years, Dr. William F. Lorenz, became clinical director of the Wisconsin State Hospital at Mendota. He looked more like a successful football coach than one to lead us to important public health steps in reducing the incidence of syphilis and into a broader understanding of neuropsychiatric problems. He was a big man, an athlete who weighed close to two hundred pounds and who had played a line position successfully while a college student and had won prizes as a weight lifter. Lorenz was a large man in many senses of the word, with broad interests, compelling enthusiasms, and a deep resonant voice that aroused attention anywhere. His manifest sincerity and conviction was a bid to good cheer whether he was pleading for his causes before legislative committees, or merely saying good morning to you at the University Club. He was fundamentally interested in his fellow man, especially those with serious and possibly preventable disease handicaps.

William F. Lorenz was born February 15, 1882, in Brooklyn, New York, and died February 19, 1958, in Madison, Wisconsin. He was attending the public schools of New York city when the Spanish-American War broke out. He was caught up, as were so many young men, in the emotional excitement of the war. He left school without ceremony; although only sixteen, he was large for his age and he succeeded in some way in enlisting in the volunteer army. He never lost his enthusiasm for athletics and for the military.

Returning to New York after the war, he went to Trinity School and then to New York University–Bellevue Hospital Medical College, obtaining his M.D. degree in 1903. As a medical student, our athlete earned some of his expenses by singing in church choirs, notably Episcopal. His postgraduate interest was psychiatry, with training at the Manhattan State Hospital. In 1908, he joined a group of psychiatrists at Kankakee, Illinois, to work chiefly with Dr. Adolph Meyer, who later became the distinguished professor of neuropsychiatry at Johns Hopkins University. While visiting in Wisconsin, Lorenz became interested in the opportunities offered in psychiatry by Wisconsin's mental health program and its state institutions.

Earlier, in 1907, Dr. Charles Gorst, then superintendent of Wisconsin State Hospital (now Mendota State Hospital), had recommended a ten-year plan for the development of that institution. One part of the plan provided for a department of research, with a neuropathologist to serve also in the medical department of the University and hold class clinics in the hospital; space and equipment were to be furnished by the University for a laboratory for research work on mental and nervous diseases, and the pathologist's salary was to be paid by the Board of Control.

The Board was unable to obtain a neuropathologist, and much of this suggested plan was not realized for years.

The Board did appreciate, however, that an active laboratory could be of service to all state institutions, so they clung to that idea, and by resolution, designated this research laboratory as the Wisconsin Psychiatric Institute. In Dr. Lorenz they had a man who, although not a neuropathologist by formal training, enjoyed laboratory work,[1] always emphasized post-mortem studies, and was vitally interested in creating a diagnostic center for the mentally ill and a research institution to observe and study the problems of the patients in our Wisconsin institutions. Thus, in 1914 Lorenz was appointed the first director of the Wisconsin Psychiatric Institute. In defining the Institute, Lorenz wrote: "The purpose of the Institute is to assist in the care and treatment of the insane and any other wards of the state in whom mental or physical diseases bring about their state care. This assistance is to be rendered by scientific research work. The investigations are primarily directed toward the cause of conditions that result in state care."[2]

Dr. Lorenz's personal association with members of the University of Wisconsin Medical School faculty gave opportunity for cooperative research. This was recognized by his appointment in 1915 as associate professor of psychiatry without pay. His collaboration with Dr. Arthur S. Loevenhart and the changing group working with experimental syphilis was highly productive.

Years of work by Dr. Loevenhart and his associates on biological oxidation with detailed studies of respiratory stimulation in experimental animals came to dramatic fruition through cooperation with Dr. Lorenz, who by his position in the Wisconsin Psychiatric Institute had medical contact with completely hopeless psychotic cases. Initially, in 1918, ten cases, most of them diagnosed as dementia paralytica, were treated with dilute sodium cyanide injected intravenously. The report of the experiment states that in every case with no untoward results, "we have obtained a marked stimulation of the respiration on the average within twenty seconds after starting the injection." One case, with a diagnosis of dementia praecox, who had not spoken since he was admitted to the hospital, gave the most startling response: "Immediately following the injection he talked freely and gave a history which was later verified."[3]

World War I both slowed the regular work of the Institute and also prevented advance in these cooperative researches. A decade later, however, further studies confirmed and amplified the earlier observations. Besides sodium cyanide, which would be considered by most physicians too dangerous an agent to use, the studies showed that "a mixture of carbon dioxide and oxygen is a far better agent for producing cerebral stimulation in the stuporous phase of certain psychoses." It was reported that "by these simple chemical procedures the mental processes in certain psychotic patients are restored toward normal for a period of from two to twenty-five minutes." [4] A description of the reactions of a patient under observation and the dumbfounded surprise of the physicians in attendance will help us to relive the scene:

> The group of observers had left their seats and crowded about the stage as Dr. Ralph Waters had put the mask over the patient's face. All of a sudden, the audience was electrified as the patient sat up and shouted, "What are all these people doing here?" Waving her arms, she screamed, "Go back, go back." . . . The visitors as one man fell back upon each other, startled, and amazed.[5]

It has been commonly conceded that these experiments were one of the most important and well-received pieces of work in this field in the United States, opening up the whole concept of shock therapy with agents other than electrical devices. This was a forerunner of present-day tranquilizers.

Soon after World War I, in 1919, the staff of the Institute became a part of a research group in association with pharmacology and other departments. Through the hospital facilities of the Institute, the arsenicals that had given successful indications in laboratory studies were tried on human patients with notable success.

In 1924, with the building of the Wisconsin General Hospital and the beginning of the complete medical course, Dr. Lorenz earnestly recommended that the Psychiatric Institute be transferred to and be made part of the medical department of the University of Wisconsin: "The research activities of this Institute are medical and educational. These have been possible in large part because of the close affiliations maintained with the scientific departments of the state university. . . ." [6] In 1925 this recommendation was approved by the legislature and the Institute was transferred from Mendota to Madison and became an integral part of the University and the neuropsychiatry department of the Medical School. A page from the University catalogue summarizes the story well:

WISCONSIN PSYCHIATRIC INSTITUTE
W. F. Lorenz, Director, Professor of Neuropsychiatry

The Wisconsin Psychiatric Institute was developed originally under the Board of Control of the State of Wisconsin. It was started in 1915 at Mendota where research in mental and nervous disorders was carried on. On July 1, 1925 the Wisconsin Psychiatric Institute was transferred to the University by the legislature. Its primary purpose was preserved. The transfer to the University afforded increased opportunities in research through cooperation with the departments of the medical school and other departments of the University. Basically, the program is designed to initiate and promote measures of relief and prevention in the field of neuropsychiatry, more especially as mental and nervous disorders become problems for the state and communities.

The earliest research activities of the Institute centered about syphilis, and in cooperation with the State Board of Health much has been accomplished in the course of thirty years. At Wisconsin the Institute pioneered in providing free blood and spinal fluid examinations to the physicians, institutions, and hospitals of the State. At a later date the Institute provided a service in blood chemistry on the same basis. In cooperation with the department of pharmacology the staff of the Institute undertook extensive research in the field of treatment, especially syphilis. New drugs were developed and the experimental phases of such research were carried on by the staff of the Institute in cooperation with the department of pharmacology. After about twenty years of service in testing blood, during which time approximately one-third of the population of the State of Wisconsin was tested as a routine procedure when sick, the incidence of syphilis in Wisconsin was definitely known. It was also known to what degree syphilis was responsible for mental and nervous disorders in the State of Wisconsin. In 1937, the legislature passed an act requiring all applicants for marriage licenses to have a blood test for syphilis. In 1940, as military preparedness began, blood testing for syphilis of recruits and selectees became an additional service by the Institute laboratory. From the period of 1935–1947 inclusive, a total of 2,904,245 individuals from the State of Wisconsin were tested for syphilis. During the period from 1937–1947 433,388 persons applying for a marriage license were tested for syphilis; 451,802 persons coming under the Selective Service provisions were tested for syphilis. In short, the serological service by the laboratory division of the Wisconsin Psychiatric Institute has grown and become a very large state service in the field of public health.

During a period of years new serological techniques have been developed and more refined laboratory service to the clinician has been achieved. Among these is a rapid reliable flocculation test and also a quantitative procedure which adds to the value of blood tests for syphilis.

During the period 1915–1925, the mental disorders due to syphilis cared for at our state institutions amounted to approximately 12% of the admission rate. This rate was similar to that found in other midwestern states. During the last fifteen years the rate has decreased approximately 3%. An extensive survey made by the U.S. Public Health Service in 1940 showed Wisconsin to have the lowest rate of syphilis found in the entire United States excepting one New England state.

The staff of the Institute comprises also the staff of the department of neuropsychiatry, the university medical school, and the Wisconsin State General Hospital. Research has been stressed and carried on in such fields as encephalography, shock therapy, the use of barbiturates in the treatment of mental disorders and in methods of examination. As a by-product of certain of these investigations an antidote for barbiturate poisoning was developed. Space does not permit a detailed account of the constant research and investigation that is being carried on.

The Institute operates in three divisions: diagnostic laboratory service; medical education; clinical or hospital service in connection with the Wisconsin State General Hospital. All divisions are used in the program of medical education for students, interns, residents, and visiting physicians. The purpose of the Institute is more fully realized by its administration as a department of the University in close affiliation with the medical school and the Wisconsin State General Hospital.[7]

The professorial staff of the newly constituted department of neuropsychiatry in the Wisconsin Medical School, and its other parent, the Psychiatric Institute, included Drs. William F. Lorenz, William J. Bleckwenn, and Hans H. Reese. This group of physicians was unusual in several respects — for their athletic prowess and military service, for the variety of their interests, for their successful united and individual attacks on syphilis and related problems, and for their ready collaboration with members of other departments.[8]

With well-defined subdivision of the responsibilities, so that each member of the staff followed his special interest while all joined forces in the major drive, the group and each individual of the group made splendid contributions. Lorenz was in charge of the laboratory studies and worked intensively with Loevenhart and associates. To Dr. Bleckwenn was given responsibility for the trial of various arsenicals and later the barbiturates. Dr. Reese's field of study as an especially competent neurologist was damage to the autonomic nervous system and the effects of various drugs on this system. After Wagner-Jauregg's discovery of the therapeutic value of malaria inoculation had been confirmed, Dr. Reese introduced this form of treatment in Mendota hospital. The tertian strain passed from patient to patient became a basis for cooperative study with the Mayo Clinic and with the several Chicago medical schools.[9]

These men would be the first to testify that much of their success was due to scientific advances international in origin, providing knowledge of the syphilitic nature of previously obscure diseases and better means of therapy. In these broad fields, they published well over a hundred papers. Tryparsamide, which was found of value in rabbit syphilis by Loevenhart and associates, was proved by Lorenz and collaborators to be highly valuable in the treatment of syphilis chiefly of the central nervous system.[10] It was, perhaps, the most effective agent in this condition until the rise of penicillin replaced earlier pharmacological treatments.

The investigations of various sedatives culminated in the use of sodium amytal to assay commonly unapproachable mental conflicts. This type of analysis found extensive application during World War II in the restoration of psychologically induced battle casualties.[11]

At the centennial anniversary of the foundation of the American Psychiatric Association, Drs. Lorenz and Bleckwenn were given credit for the introduction of sodium amytal as a suitable drug to release inhibitions and to uncover suppressed memories. Menninger gives credit to Bleckwenn for first using sodium amytal for prolonged narcosis and as a method for obtaining information from mute psychotic patients and to Roy Grinker and associates for developing "narcosynthesis." He said, "A majority of American psychiatrists preferred sodium pentothal over any other drug."[12]

Dr. Reese says that Dr. Lorenz injected an exploratory spirit into all the Institute group so that their investigations covered many areas of medicine and public weal that cannot even be suggested in this brief story of the whole Wisconsin Medical School. One wonders how this rather earthy man, Dr. Lorenz, with his frequently self-centered enthusiasms came to stress that your enemies or infections are my enemies and therefore the responsibility of the public.[13] Of course, this point of view was apparent to seers in Biblical times and even before. This attitude became more general after the rise of bacteriology in the last quarter of the nineteenth and the first quarter of the twentieth century.

Lorenz's breadth of interest is further suggested by papers on pellagra made when the successful study of this disease by Goldberger and associates was in its infancy (1914). Lorenz's group of pellagrins was too small for any conclusions, but most of the patients fed on a generous high protein diet did show improvement, thus adding a small bit to the dietary deficiency concept of the disease.[14]

As a lover of the out-of-doors, Dr. Lorenz took an active interest in sports and was for eleven years a member of the University athletic board and its chairman during many of these years. He was an enthusiast in whatever he undertook, but was inclined to lose interest after the initial urge and excitement. As a boy he had sailed the waters of Long Island

Sound, and boating was one hobby in which his interest never flagged. During his life he built some twenty-five craft of many sizes and types and frequently did a considerable portion of the work with his own hands. The largest was a two-masted schooner, the Sea Gull, that sailed the blue waters of Lake Mendota.

Few members of our faculty have left Madison with the warm appreciation and affection of so many as did Bill Bleckwenn when he was granted leave of absence for serious ill health in 1954 and journeyed to the warmer climate of Winter Haven, Florida. His hope for recovery was not fully realized, and although he came back to Madison occasionally, he never again took up his full professorial duties.

His brief return for the dedication of the neurology library and the presentation of a Medical School chair to Dr. Reese on September 23, 1964, is a happy memory. Another cherished memory — not so happy from the world point of view, but a picture which both family and friends carry engraved in their minds — is that of Bill in his full vigor and effectiveness when he returned as an officer of the medical corps about 1940, fresh from the early maneuvers in Texas. He declared that the troops were fit; he himself certainly looked that part completely.

Dr. William Jefferson Bleckwenn was born in Astoria, New York, July 23, 1895, and died on January 6, 1965, in Winter Haven, Florida. He received his secondary education in the public schools of New York, his B.S. degree, including the first two years of medicine, at Wisconsin in 1915–17, and his M.D. degree from the College of Physicians and Surgeons, Columbia University, in 1920. His powerful and graceful body gave him opportunities in the heavier field sports in college; he did well in putting the shot, in hurling the discus.

After residencies at Bellevue Hospital, New York, and the Wisconsin Psychiatric Institute, Dr. Bleckwenn became instructor at the Institute in 1922. His responsibilities and rank in the department of neuropsychiatry and the Institute advanced with his increasing competence and knowledge. He attained the title of assistant director of the Institute. He became an associate professor in 1930 and a full professor in 1934, serving continuously save for leave of absence during World War II, until serious cardiovascular illness forced him to retire.

As a teacher Dr. Bleckwenn was known for his pungent phraseology; as an administrator he was superior; as a psychiatrist, he was devoted to his patients and effective both at the bedside and in his research. He also gave much energy to committee work and to community services in mental health. His introduction of the use of sodium amytal in the drug therapy of psychiatry was a real advance. With Dr. Mabel Masten he demonstrated the effectiveness of picrotoxin as a satisfactory antidote in barbiturate intoxication.[15]

Dr. Hans H. Reese, recently arrived from his native country, Germany, climbed down from the train at the old railroad station (now destroyed) at Mendota, Wisconsin, at 1:10 P.M. on a Friday in September, 1924, and was met by the "hotel keeper, postmaster, chief of police and storekeeper — same man, with a model T. Ford touring car." After Reese had met with the chief, Dr. Lorenz, Bleckwenn took the new appointee around to meet the staff of the Psychiatric Institute, "who were taking their noon siesta (playing Kelly pool) in the Soldiers' Memorial recreation hut adjoining the W.P.I." Later that afternoon the World Series baseball game was being broadcast over radio, and although Dr. Reese had never seen a baseball game he was canny enough to wager that Babe Ruth would make a home run every time he came to the bat. "The Babe made three that day and Hans collected royally from all of us." [16] And then his new colleagues took off for a hunting expedition. Wasn't that a typical and familiar introduction to these United States and to the Wisconsin Psychiatric Institute?

Reese was born in Bordesholm, Germany, September 17, 1891. He obtained his medical degree from the University of Kiel, Germany, in 1917. He served as assistant surgeon in the German navy, 1917–18. After that, he worked for five years at the University of Hamburg, as assistant in internal medicine, in pathology, and in neuropsychiatry, obtaining a broad foundation in internal medicine as well as in neurology, the specialty in which he has since contributed so successfully. After his arrival at the Wisconsin Psychiatric Institute in 1924 and the combining of the Institute with the University of Wisconsin Medical School, he enjoyed many years of effective medical practice, teaching, and research in the fields of his choice, establishing a well-merited reputation for medical wisdom and human interest and generosity. He became a naturalized citizen of the United States in 1929. He gladly accepted responsibilities, taught with a flair for dramatic demonstration and published through the years about a hundred papers, including a dozen or more in medical history. In addition to his work on syphilis, he published on schizophrenia and made important contributions to our knowledge of multiple sclerosis.

Dr. Reese's broad clinical experience and skill in diagnosis were especially valuable here in the Medical School and in the Wisconsin Psychiatric Institute. His patients were devoted to him, and he to them. In his contact with patients, as also with his friends, Dr. Reese had an Old World gracious courtesy that has been cherished by all.

The work of this trio — Lorenz, Bleckwenn, and Reese — was later ably enriched by that of two younger neuropsychiatrists, Drs. Mabel Masten and Annette Washburne.

Mabel G. Masten was born in Mineral Point, Wisconsin, December 29, 1897, and grew up in the neighboring town of Darlington. With a B.S. degree from the University of Chicago (1921) that included several courses in bacteriology she worked for a year in that field before returning to complete the work for the M.D. degree at Rush Medical College of the University of Chicago in 1925. The University of Wisconsin was at that time opening its four-year course; Dr. Masten became our first woman intern and continued earning the friendship and approval of her associates through a residency in neuropsychiatry to become an important member of that department with the well-earned recognition as professor in 1950. When her colleagues left for military service in World War II, Dr. Masten became the chairman of the department. Of her publications, that in collaboration with Dr. Bleckwenn on the antidotal treatment of barbiturate with picrotoxin merits high commendation. She writes, "I did all the actual work, with Bill B. on the side lines calling the plays." She is "most proud" of her paper on neurogenic erosions of the gastrointestinal tract, which was stimulated by a remark of Dr. Middleton at an autopsy and a reference to Dr. Harvey Cushing's Balfour Lecture.[17]

Although it takes us beyond our terminal date, I must record our regret that family affairs took her away from us to Florida and the Veterans Administration in 1954. She was always so encouraging to her patients and so altogether dependable and friendly. We have all missed her.

Another of the younger members of the neuropsychiatry faculty was Dr. Annette C. Washburne, who for so many years handled some of the emotional problems and more serious psychiatric ones in student health. She was deeply interested in the family of each patient. She was born in Chicago, Illinois, October 6, 1898, graduated from DePaul University in 1925, and from the University of Illinois College of Medicine in 1929. She came to the Psychiatric Institute in 1930 and continued with the department, attaining full professorship in 1948. She left to go into private practice in 1954, beyond our period. She contributed to the physiological studies in the use of sodium amytal and also significantly to the study of the hazards of uncontrolled use of bromides.[18]

With many faculty members away at the war in 1940, Dr. Fritz Kant came from Kraepelin's clinic in Munich to be professor of neuropsychiatry here. He had had excellent psychiatric services not only in Munich but also in Tübingen and Berlin. He brought with him a fresh point of view "breaking with descriptive psychiatry, replacing it with a dynamic constitutional appraisal." He introduced some of Freud's ideas and a strong interest in mental hygiene. To the medical students he provided a new and sympathetic stimulus. At the end of the war, he continued on a part-time basis with considerable private practice well beyond our period. He published several papers on alcoholism and its treatment; these studies were brought together in a book, *The Treatment of the Alcoholic*.[19]

Both the Wisconsin Psychiatric Institute and the State Laboratory of Hygiene, already described, are excellent examples of mutually favorable cooperation on the part of different state agencies, in this case the Board of Public Welfare and the University of Wisconsin.

RESIDENTS IN NEUROPSYCHIATRY THROUGH 1950

1927	Edward McKinley
1930	Bertram G. Lawrence
1931	Annette C. Washburne
1934	E. Murray Burns
1937	Marc J. Musser
	W. A. Nosik
1938	Howard L. Correll
1939	Mark Foster
1940	Cyril A. Schwarze
1948	Andrew W. Dwyer
	Harold N. Lubing
1949	William H. Heywood
	Max M. Smith
1950	Marjorie R. Piehl

19 Department of Medicine

*In illness one should take care of two things, to do good
and not to do harm.*

Hippocrates

In June, 1945, Dr. Joseph Evans retired from the chairmanship of the department of medicine in which he had been the beloved chief for so many years. One of his excellent protégés, Dr. Ovid
Otto Meyer, who had come to the University from Stevens Point back
in 1924 and had developed admirably in the intervening years, was chosen
in his stead. Meyer took his undergraduate degree and first two years of
medical training here and completed his studies for the medical degree at
Columbia University in 1926. He returned to Wisconsin for his internship and residency in medicine. He then spent the next years, 1929–32,
at Huntington Memorial Hospital and Thorndike Laboratories in the
Harvard Medical Center, studying diseases of the blood and of the glands
of internal secretion. Upon his return to Wisconsin, he was named assistant professor of medicine and he continued his steady, productive
advancement, attaining his professorship in 1944. When Dr. Meyer took
over the important task of chairmanship of the department of medicine,
all were aware that during the pressures of the war years and Dr. Evans'
failing strength it was this younger man who had actually been carrying
the heavier burdens both in the care of patients and in teaching the
students.

Dr. Meyer's many studies on the obscure anemias and leukemias of
man amplified by his experimental work in lower animals, his studies
with Dr. Middleton on bone marrow insufficiency, his work with anticoagulants and on thrombosis, and his early use of penicillin in the treatment of sub-acute bacterial endocarditis, have advanced considerably our

135

knowledge of hematology and diseases of the blood-forming organs. In scanning his bibliography of well over seventy titles, documentation must be restricted to two or three of Meyer's favorites, on the hypophysis and hematopoiesis and studies on coumarin anticoagulants.[1]

In 1932, hematological studies were aided materially by the setting up of a special research laboratory in the department of pathology. Miss Ethel Thewlis, a native of England, trained in the offices of Drs. George Minot and William P. Murphy of Boston and by Drs. Miller and Bunting here at Wisconsin, collaborated ably with many of those working in experimental and clinical studies. An early paper with Meyer on the blood count of normal rats and one with Meyer and Middleton on leucocytosis following parenteral injection of liver extract may be cited.[2]

Dr. Meyer's critical analyses of his cases for student teaching and his warm interest in his patients have worked wonders for our students and residents in medicine and have clarified difficult questions for all the faculty. Dr. Middleton has said, "Keenly alert at the bedside, Ovid Meyer's diagnostic acumen has been the source of deep satisfaction to his associates and comfort to his patients and their families."[3]

Postgraduate medicine is being stressed by all medical schools, and we have not neglected these opportunities. With substantial funds from the Wisconsin Alumni Research Foundation, a fruitful symposium in 1939 on the blood and blood-forming organs was accorded high praise by those working in the field. The anemias and the leukemias, both in man and in experimental animals, provided the basis for the volume of the papers, for which Dr. Meyer wrote the foreword.[4]

We must, of course, point out a few of the hobbies and foibles of our leaders. Dr. Meyer enjoyed his golf, but followed the more strenuous games as an avid supporter and observer. He delighted in professional baseball records and performances, especially those of the New York Yankees. At lunch time, we all remember how he picked up wagers from anyone who scorned their prowess. Of course, Babe Ruth was his favorite player and rarely failed him. As Meyer was also an ardent Democrat, surrounded by ultra-conservative Republicans, many a discussion was supported by a gentleman's wager, and, as we all know, in recent years his party has commonly been on the winning side.

With his gay boutonniere, his prompt friendly responses to those in need, and his thoughtful answers to moot questions, Dr. Meyer has been a stimulating teacher, the physicians' physician, and an efficient leader in the most important department of the medical school. His history of the department of medicine is excellent.[5]

CARDIOLOGY

Cardiology and the knowledge of cardiovascular disease have been enriched by men and studies here at Wisconsin since the beginning of the physiology department, and these fields have continued to be the interests of a highly productive group well beyond our historical period. Dr. Eyster was our first cardiologist, presenting thus a shining example of the interweaving at that early period of our underlying science departments and clinical investigations. Eyster's fundamental studies pointed out that muscle injury resulting from initial dilatation is a necessary precursor of cardiac hypertrophy. These studies were followed by illuminating researches both by him and his successor, Dr. Chester M. Kurtz, in heart size and shape as demonstrated by X-ray methods. Dr. Kurtz published a splendid long-term study analyzing over 1700 patients by the orthodiascopic method.[6] His work with rheumatic heart disease and its prevention also merits commendation.

Dr. Kurtz was born in Wisconsin, took his undergraduate work and first two years of medical training here, completing studies for the M.D. degree at Harvard in 1927. He then came back to this university and continued to advance in stature and in the favor of his students, his patients, and his professional peers. We regret greatly his later departure from the Medical School to carry on his work in a milder climate, New Mexico. Earlier in his career, Chester Kurtz was in mathematics and engineering until he recognized some of the more human possibilities of medicine. Always, however, in his medical work we observed the sharp nicety of his approach to problems, characteristic, I assume, of the mathematician. We miss him.

Herman H. Shapiro came to us from his homeland, Russia; we are therefore in debt to that country. Here at the University he majored in economics and then switched to medicine, earning the M.D. degree here in 1932. He followed Drs. Eyster and Kurtz in cardiology with a special emphasis on Einthoven's string galvanometer methods of cardiac study.[7] Shapiro's paper demonstrating transient electrocardiographic changes during an angina attack merits our attention. His summary paper on treatment of congestive heart failure was an outgrowth of a rich symposium on that subject for the State Medical Society.[8] Dr. Shapiro's keen interest in his patients and his gracious courtesy have been much appreciated both by patients and by the faculty. His chief hobby is tied in with his love of the land; he owns a good farm not far from Madison and, when possible, takes pleasure in turning over the soil. Since he is one of the younger members of the faculty, his growing career must be left largely for a future historian to present.

An important anticoagulant, dicumarol, isolated from spoiled sweetclover hay by Karl Paul Link of the department of biochemistry, has become almost legendary as an example of experiments in pure science that proved to have astounding practical applications. Dr. Link collaborated to some degree with Dr. Ovid Meyer and other members of the department of medicine in their early application of dicumarol in the treatment of heart cases.[9]

DERMATOLOGY

As mentioned earlier, Dr. Otto Hottinger Foerster (1876–1965), our first professor of dermatology, came to Madison regularly one day each week from Milwaukee, beginning in 1925. He gave generously of his experience and skill, building up a happy, productive department and association until his official retirement in 1946. The division of dermatology should be cited as one that has been highly successful and productive with its staff on a part-time basis.

Foerster was one of the early specialists in dermatology in this country. Before joining our staff, he had had wide experience in Philadelphia (M.D., University of Pennsylvania, 1898) and also in Vienna. He became one of the founders of Columbia Hospital, Milwaukee, and was chief of staff there for ten years and dermatologist for fifty years.

One of his younger associates, Dr. Garrett Cooper, says that his lectures were stereotyped and uninteresting, but that it was a delight to watch him examine a patient. He was meticulous and exacting, starting at the scalp, inspecting the ears, the eyebrows, and the skin very closely. Occasionally he would remove one pair of glasses and put on a pair of pince-nez, which gave him a magnified view of the skin lesions. He would then back off and consider, and then re-examine the patient before he made any decisions. Dr. Foerster used the X-ray early in his practice. He noted that many of the men using the rays placed their hands between the beam and the fluoroscopic screen to adjust the voltage and intensity of the rays. Responding to a question from Dr. Cooper as to how he avoided the severe burns so common among his early associates in dermatology, Dr. Foerster replied, "I was afraid of the damn stuff." He developed a graduated lead shield, which he introduced into the beam by means of a handle, so that his hands were never exposed and remained excellent to the end of his practice when he was well along into his eighties.

Foerster was a prolific contributor to the general medical journals and to those of his specialty and published articles on X-ray injuries, the use of radium in dermatology, and a considerable number of papers on the treatment of syphilis, as well as chapters in major textbooks. A noteworthy contribution with a number of his younger associates stemmed from studies in the department of pharmacology by Tatum and Cooper in the use of Mapharsen in experimental syphilis.[10] Following the apparent improvement in experimental syphilitic rabbits after treatment with Mapharsen, Dr. Tatum turned a quantity of the drug over to Dr. Foerster, who tried it on patients both in Milwaukee and in Madison. Many patients showed a favorable response. The work was carried out, as Cooper says, so meticulously, and the clinical conclusions were so accurate, that no change has been necessary in any of the observations made by the group here and in Milwaukee.[11]

As Dr. Foerster grew older, he gradually gave up his weekly trips to Madison, turning over the responsibilities here to his associates, Drs. McIntosh and Cooper.

Dr. Roscoe Lyle McIntosh (1891–1952), a native of Wisconsin, received his undergraduate and his first two years of medical instruction at the University; he received his medical degree from Washington University in 1921. He interned at Wisconsin General Hospital, specialized in dermatology at Barnard Skin and Cancer Hospital, St. Louis, and at the London School of Dermatology before returning here in 1924 to be Dr. Foerster's chief associate. He remained on a part-time basis and in private practice throughout his life. In addition to his work in dermatology, McIntosh took courses in the Wisconsin Law School in order to give to our students a course in medical jurisprudence. His published papers were mostly written with Dr. Foerster and other members of the department. A paper on the favorable results following the use of Mapharsen in Vincent's infection may be cited.[12]

Dr. McIntosh's "patience and his fine sense of Scottish humor made his teaching practical and his practice worthwhile. He was greatly interested in the athletic activities of the University, especially in the boxing teams." [13]

Dr. Garrett Arthur Cooper, one of our younger men in dermatology, tells pleasant tales of his associations with Dr. Foerster. Cooper had excellent early training in pharmacology before he went into dermatology. For several years, beginning in 1928, while still carrying on his regular studies in the College of Letters and Science, Cooper worked as a research assistant — first with Loevenhart and later with Tatum and their ever-changing group of young associates — using several arsenicals in experimental trypanosomiasis, and also in experimental syphilis. Cooper received an advanced degree in pharmacology here in 1933 and his medical degree in 1935. Further work for three years in dermatology at Western Reserve Medical School preceded his return to Wisconsin. He has continued beyond our period in the department of dermatology on a part-time basis and in private practice with high success.

In 1946, when Dr. Middleton came back from the wars, Dr. Sture A. M. Johnson was appointed full-time professor of dermatology. His earlier undergraduate training and his medical degree came from the University of Oregon (M.D., 1938), where he later specialized in dermatology. He continued in this field for five years at the University of Michigan before coming to Wisconsin. Two papers, one in experimental syphilis and the other on a rare, hereditary, skin disease, suggest the breadth of his interests.[14] Dr. Johnson says of his hobbies — golf and curling — that they provide physical activity both for summer and for winter.

RESIDENTS IN DERMATOLOGY THROUGH 1950

1948	William C. Miller
1949	Charles W. Stoops
1950	James W. Bringe

GASTROENTEROLOGY

Dr. Ray Carrington Blankinship was the first member of the department of medicine to specialize in the field of gastroenterology. He was born in Naruna, Virginia, July 31, 1890; he died prematurely August 23, 1932, at the age of forty-two. Blankinship studied at the Virginia Polytechnic Institute and later at the Medical College of Virginia, where he received his medical degree in 1914. After an internship, two years in private practice, and war service from 1917–19, he came to Wisconsin, became interested in our needs in gastroenterology, and continued throughout his life to specialize in that field. Studies on classification of diseases of the colon and the gall bladder, management of peptic ulcer cases and non-specific chronic colitis became his major research interests.[15]

The students appreciated Dr. Blankinship as a teacher, especially because of his habit of analyzing each case, trying to reduce the complex problems to simpler terms, showing them how his own mind worked in ferreting out the medical diagnoses. In one man he gave us a fine example of the art and the science of medicine. He was gradually advanced in rank until at the time of his death he was associate professor of clinical medicine. As a hobby he enjoyed golf, but he always longed for the riding opportunities of the horse country of his youth in Virginia. His gay and fresh approach to life endeared him to all.

Dr. Karver L. Puestow, a native of Wisconsin, took his undergraduate studies and first two years of medical training here and the clinical years at the University of Minnesota, where he earned his medical degree in 1922. He promptly joined the staff of our department of medicine and became closely associated with Dr. Evans. Following Dr. Blankinship's death, Dr. Puestow took charge of gastroenterology and attained full professorship in 1944. His observation on the multiple functions of bacteria in the gastrointestinal tract present an especially broad understanding of the complex ecological philosophies involved.[16] With Dr. Otto Foerster, he gave a detailed account of one of the first cases of maduromycosis in this area.[17] After the earlier years, when each physician handled outpatients in his own office, Puestow began another of his many functions — the organization of the outpatient department, which has grown into such an important branch both of service and of teaching.

We all recognize that one of Dr. Evans' mantles — namely his skill in understanding and working with members of the legislature — fell on Dr. Puestow's shoulders. He instinctively seems to understand the diverse pressures under which the legislators are striving to serve all the people of the state. He has realized that although a suggestion may come from others, the initiative properly belongs with the legislature. Dr. Puestow's happy relations with the legislators helped us in obtaining the Bardeen Laboratories.

Dr. Frank L. Weston, whose personal history will be found later in this chapter, was also active in gastroenterology after Dr. Blankinship's death, and with Puestow took over the major responsibilities of the outpatient service.

METABOLIC DISEASES

Dr. Elmer L. Sevringhaus has enjoyed so many different phases in his long, active life that it is difficult to present his story briefly with sufficient emphasis on the Wisconsin periods and at the same time with satisfactory appreciation of the full years after he left us in 1946. Born in New Albany, Indiana, February 9, 1894, he received both his B.A. (1916) and M.A. (1918) degrees at Wisconsin. He was a member of the Chemical Warfare Service stationed in Science Hall, 1917–18. Characteristic of that war period, he was carrying on under S.A.T.C. status, teaching physiological chemistry, and studying medicine all at the same time.

After receiving his medical degree from Harvard in 1921, he returned to Wisconsin and continued teaching and research in the department of physiological chemistry for about six years. Then for nineteen years he carried on his studies and teaching in the department of medicine, advancing to a full professorship in 1938. He states that he will always remain grateful for the patience with which Dr. Middleton taught him more of the art and science of clinical medicine. He has a similar feeling of warm appreciation towards Dr. Joseph Evans:

Dr. Evans was wonderfully fatherly and generous to me. He personally made possible for me the study of estrogenic hormone therapy for the menopause, using his private patients and friends. In many ways, I am most proud of that paper. . . . It was actually the first clinical report published about the use of quantitatively standardized estrogens for human therapy.[18]

Of his many studies on vitamins, he cherishes especially one made in the prison at Waupun, Wisconsin, with the help of the warden, Mr. Burke, "The minimum ascorbic acid need of adults." [19]

In Dr. Sevringhaus' complete bibliography of about 140 titles extending over many areas of physiologic chemistry and medicine, we find numerous penetrating articles on diabetes and other diseases of the glands of internal secretion, a field that was his major interest for years. Steroid hormones, vitamins, and broad studies in nutrition also drew his keen attention. Eight monographs and books have come from his pen, including a highly commended *Guide for Diabetics* (eleven editions) and a "best seller," *Endocrine Therapy in General Practice*, now in its sixth edition.[20] His twelve years as director of research at the American Hoffmann-LaRoche laboratories, and his years as head of several nutrition clinics, including that at Columbia University, show the broad interests and achievements of Dr. Sevringhaus and the recognition accorded him by his peers.

Both students and faculty here at Wisconsin remember with appreciation Dr. Sevringhaus' lucid presentations in the involved fields of his concern. He was especially skillful in adapting his presentations to enlighten but not to confuse persons of varying levels of biochemical knowledge. In recent years, his international leanings and delight in travel in foreign lands have been successfully combined with his knowledge of nutrition. He has given advisory aid to several undernourished peoples.

Dr. Edgar Stillwell Gordon followed the path of progression set by Dr. Elmer Sevringhaus — first underlying training with Dr. Harold Bradley in physiological chemistry, then medical training here and at Harvard (M.D., 1932). Two years of service, one at Billings Hospital, University of Chicago, and one at Massachusetts General Hospital, gave him the clinical background for appointments here in student health and in medicine, where he has specialized in diseases of metabolism and of the glands of internal secretion. Metabolic diseases such as thyrotoxicosis, diabetes, and those involving steroid hormones occupied much of his energetic attention up to 1950. He was editor of an attractive symposium on steroid hormones in 1950, made possible through funds from the Wisconsin Alumni Research Foundation and the National Research Council. Gordon's musical temperament and training have given him effective hobbies, cello, piano and voice, which have been richly rewarding to himself, his family, and his friends.

PEDIATRICS

Manifestly, the important medical specialty of pediatrics was not needed in dealing with early student health problems, so that it was not until 1919 when Bardeen and Evans, with the strong support of Governor Philipp, succeeded in gaining legislative approval of the four-year medical school that attention could be turned in this direction. The Bradley Memorial Hospital (1920) was planned for the study and care of the diseases of infants and young children so that it gave both the urge and the opportunity to emphasize pediatrics.

Dr. John E. Gonce, born October 17, 1893, in Elkton, Maryland, came here in 1919 from the University of Pennsylvania School of Medicine and the Hospital of the University of Pennsylvania as instructor in clinical medicine. Since the growing opportunities in pediatrics attracted him, he obtained leave of absence without pay and spent the years 1922–24 at the Children's Hospital of Pennsylvania and at the children's division of the Johns Hopkins Hospital to prepare himself for his specialty.

On his return to Madison, at the time of the opening of the Wisconsin General Hospital, he was placed in charge of the division of pediatrics. With his own development and the increasing needs of the Medical School and the community, he rose in position to become our first professor of pediatrics in 1932. He continued as effective head of that subject until his untimely death at the age of sixty-two on March 25, 1956.[21]

He was such a friendly person. He made warm contacts with his little patients, their parents, and his colleagues. His skill, interest, and directness of approach to medical and personal problems secured their confidence in him as physician and adviser. His engaging, beguiling smile relieved many difficult situations.

He was an exacting teacher, with a clarity of expression in his demonstrations at the bedside and from the platform that made for excellence. He stressed practical points for the private practice of pediatrics. He persistently continued his own learning processes. When new laboratory methods were developed, he went back into the laboratory to learn for himself the techniques and limitations of the procedures.

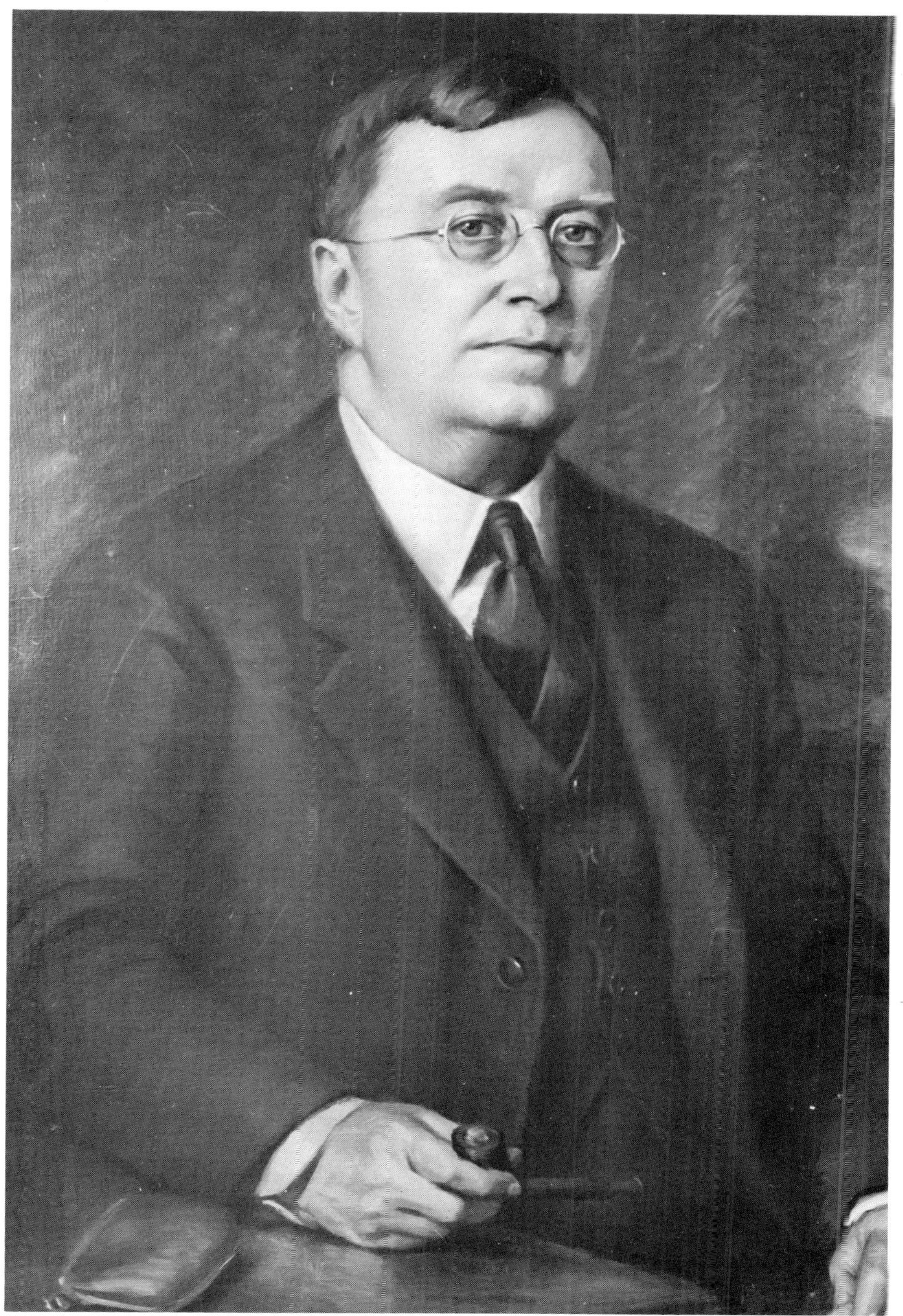

Charles Russell Bardeen, 1871–1935. First dean of the Medical School; professor of anatomy. Portrait by Herton Grenhagen.

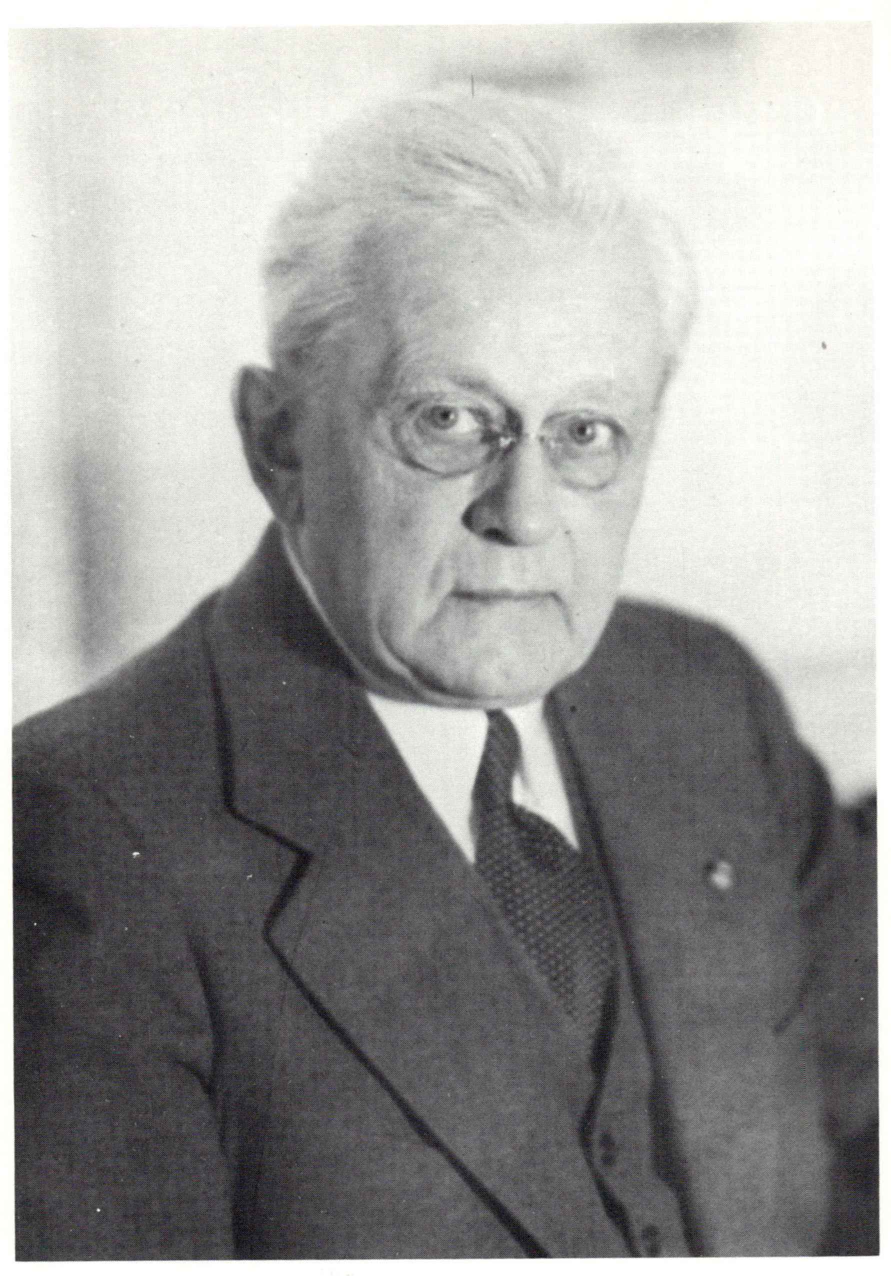

Joseph Spragg Evans, 1875–1948. First director of student health;
first professor and chairman of the department of medicine.

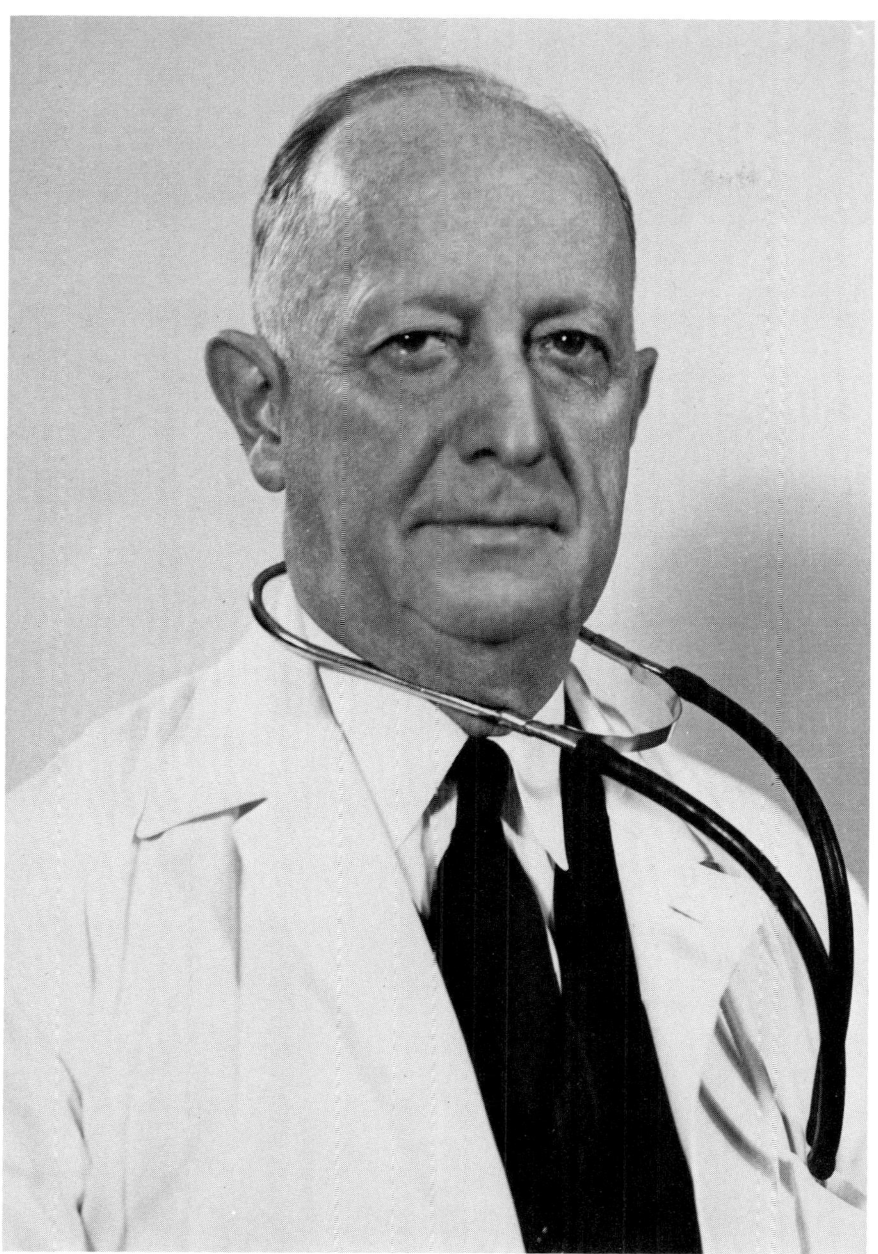

William Shainline Middleton, 1890– . Second dean of the Medical School; professor cf medicine.

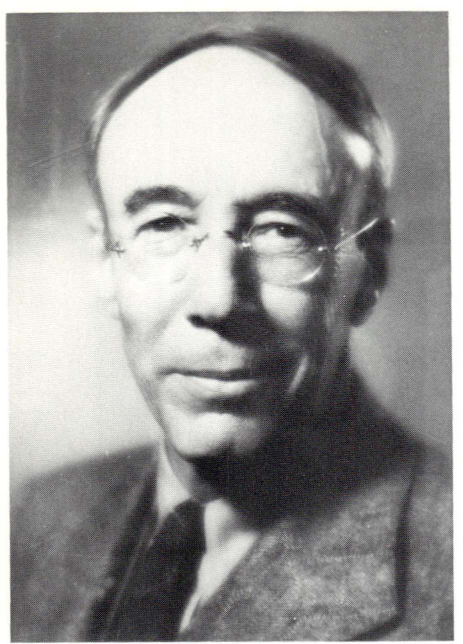

Harold Cornelius Bradley, 1878–

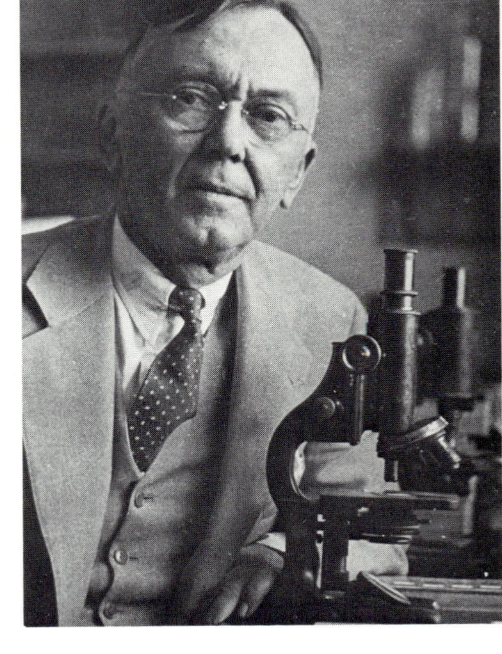

Charles Henry Bunting, 1875–1961

Edgar John Witzemann,
1884–1947

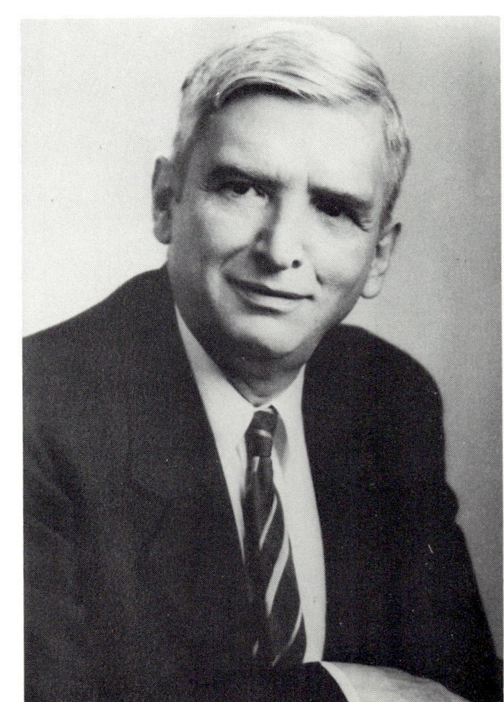

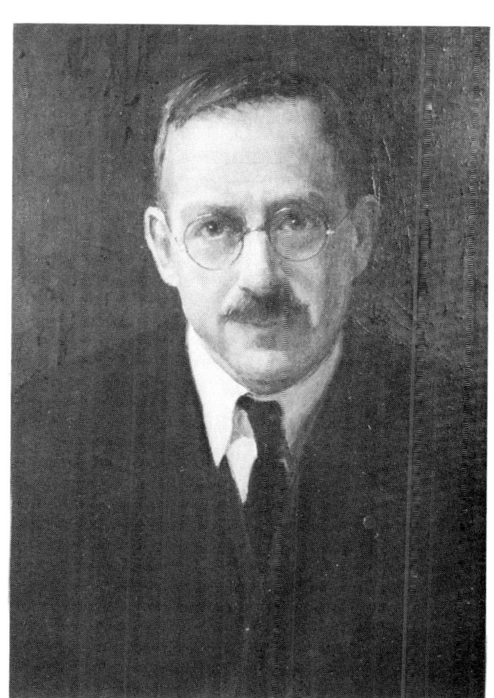

Arthur Solomon Loevenhart, 1878–1929.
Portrait by Roland Stebbins.

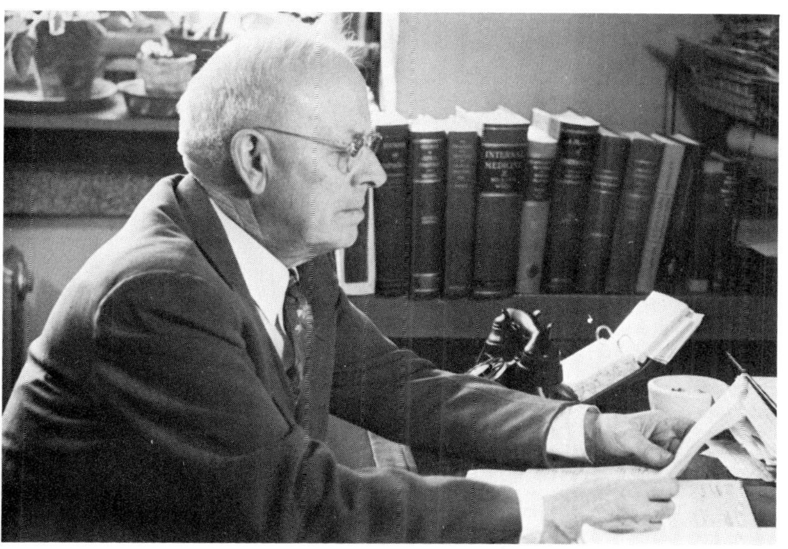

Arthur Lawrie Tatum, 1884–1955

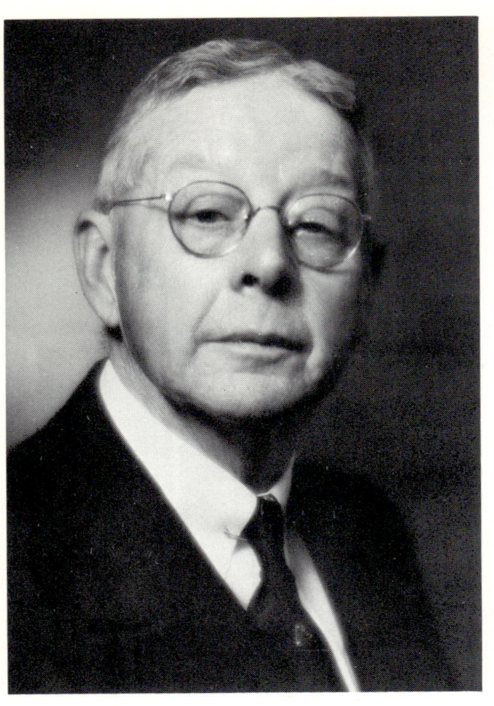

Walter Joseph Meek, 1878–1963

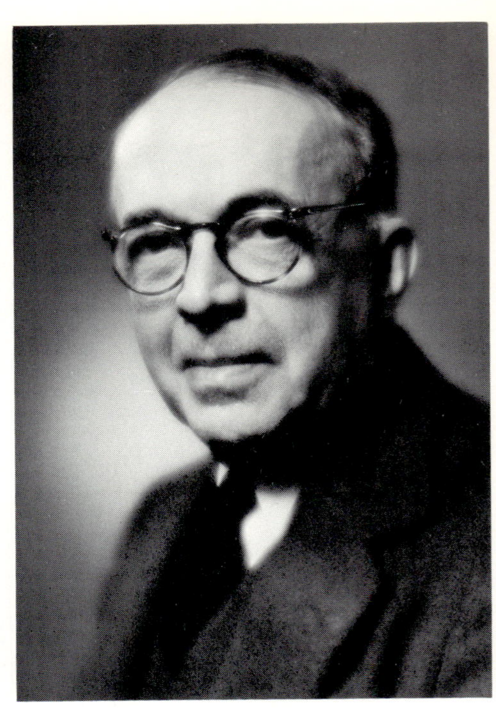

John Augustine English Eyster, 1881–1960

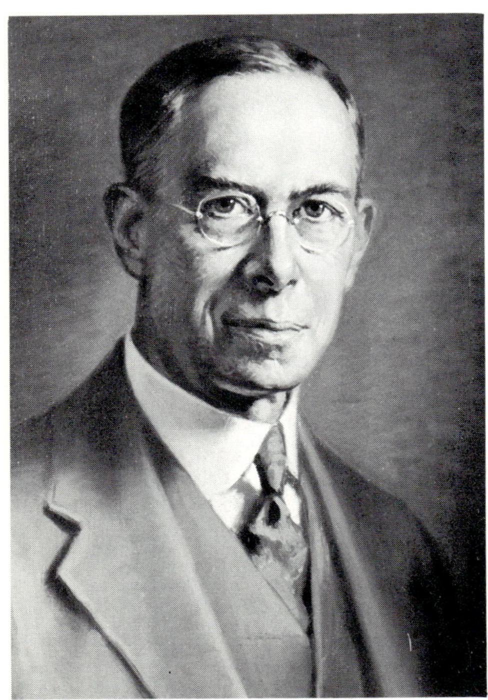

Joseph Erlanger, 1874–1965.
Portrait by Herton Grenhagen.

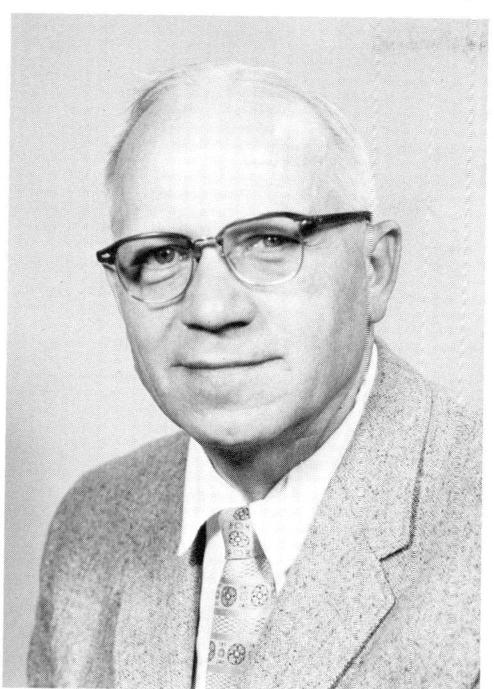

Otto Axel Mortensen, 1902–

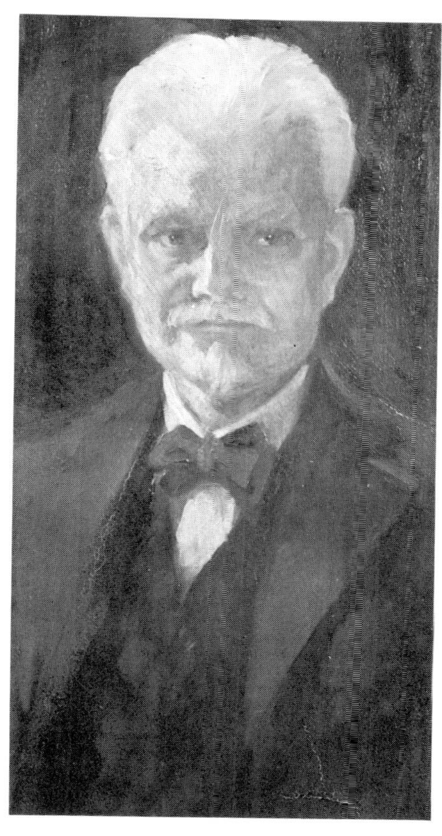

William Snow Miller, 1858–1939.
Portrait by Christian Abrahamsen.

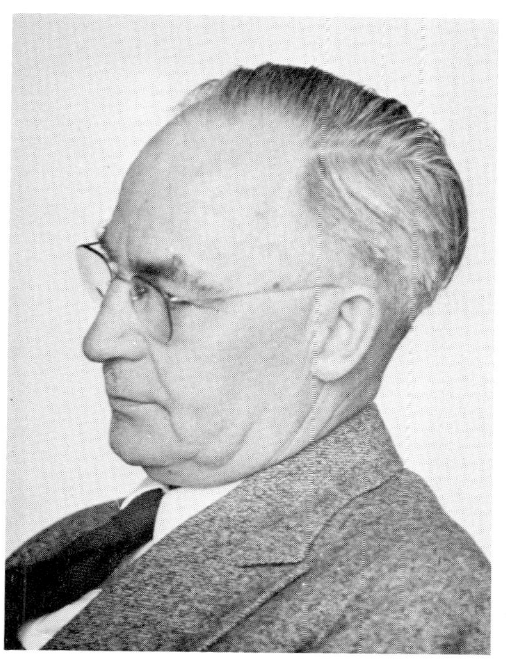

Walter Edward Sullivan, 1885–

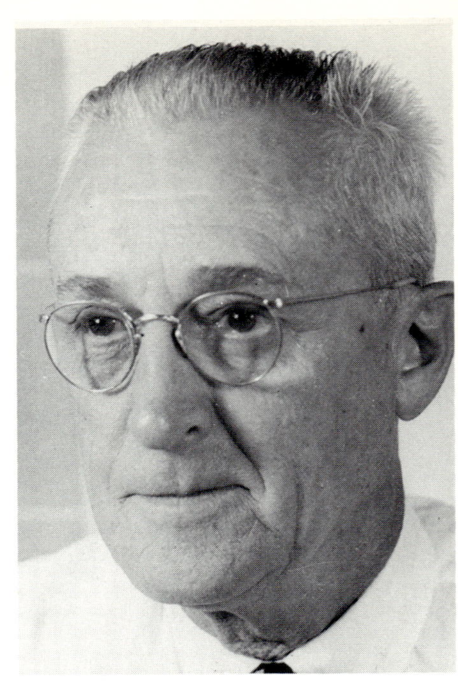

Frederick Denkmar Geist,
1895–

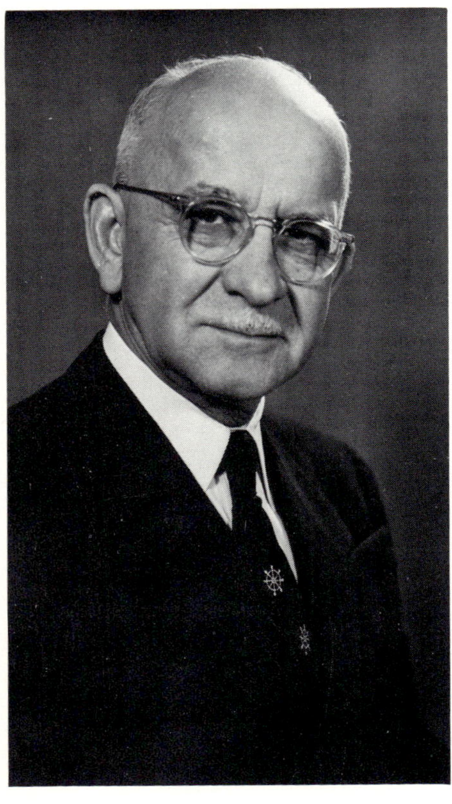

Theodore Hieronymus Bast,
1890–1959

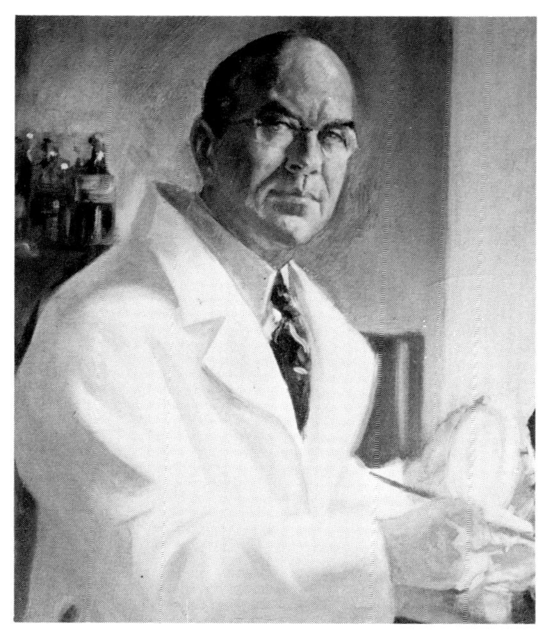

Paul Franklin Clark, 1882–.
Portrait by Myron Nutting.

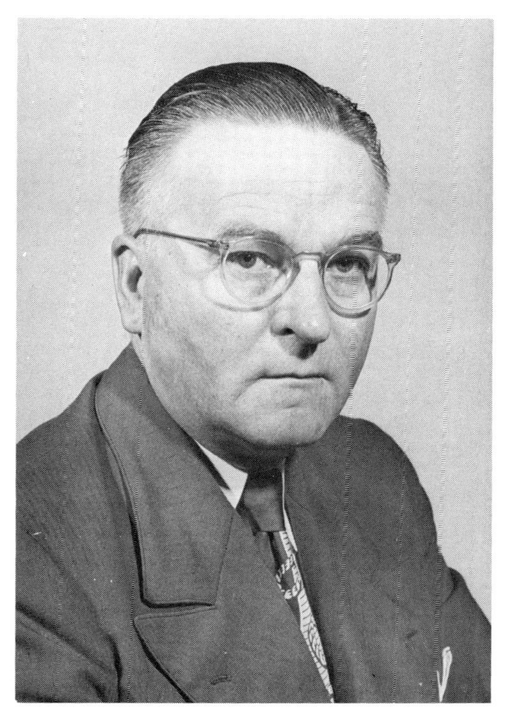

Karver Louis Puestow, 1897–

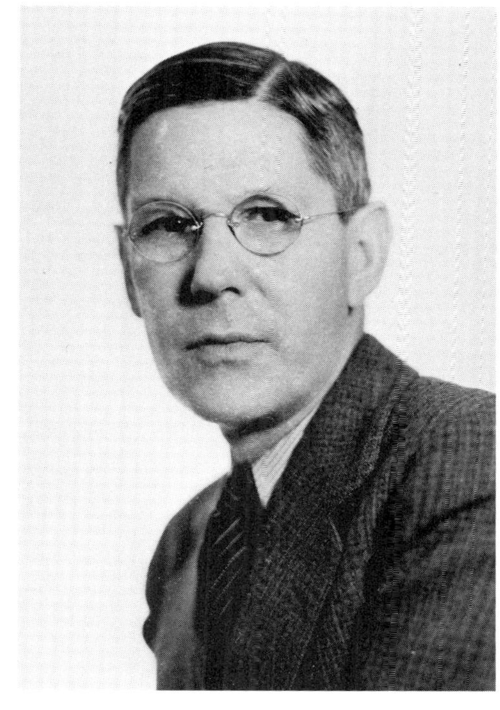

William Davidson Stovall, 1887–

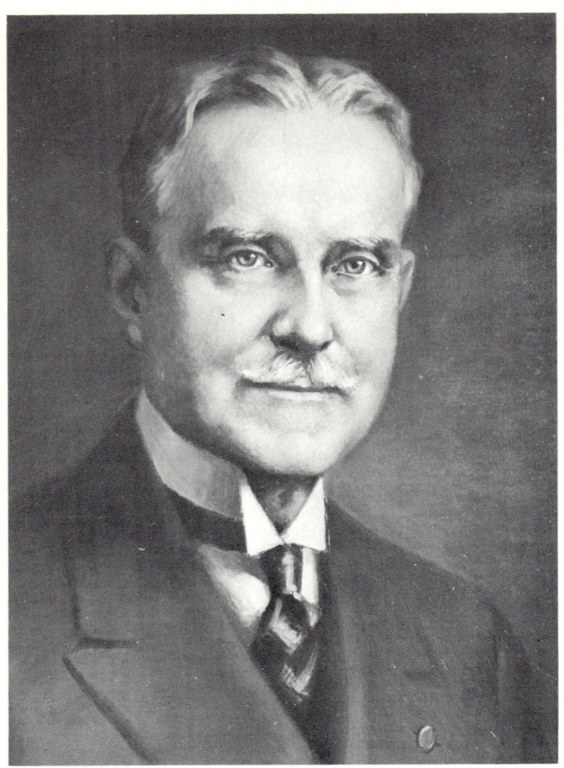

George Van Ingen Brown, 1862–194
Portrait by Herton Grenhagen.

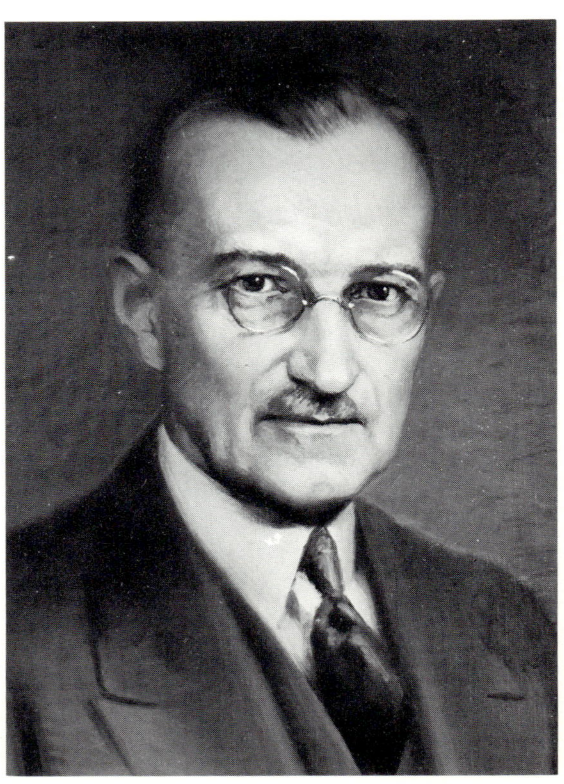

Otto Hottinger Foerster, 1876–1965.
Portrait by Herton Grenhagen.

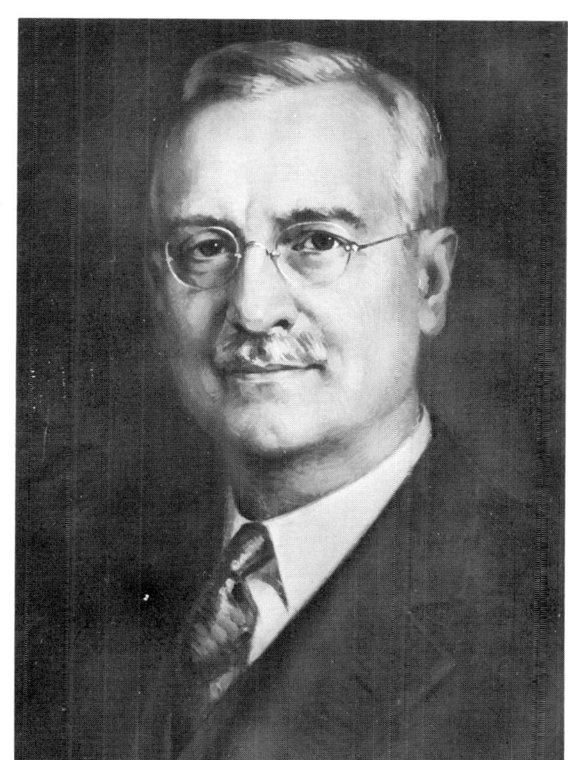

ederick Julius Gaenslen, 1877–1937.
Portrait by Herton Grenhagen.

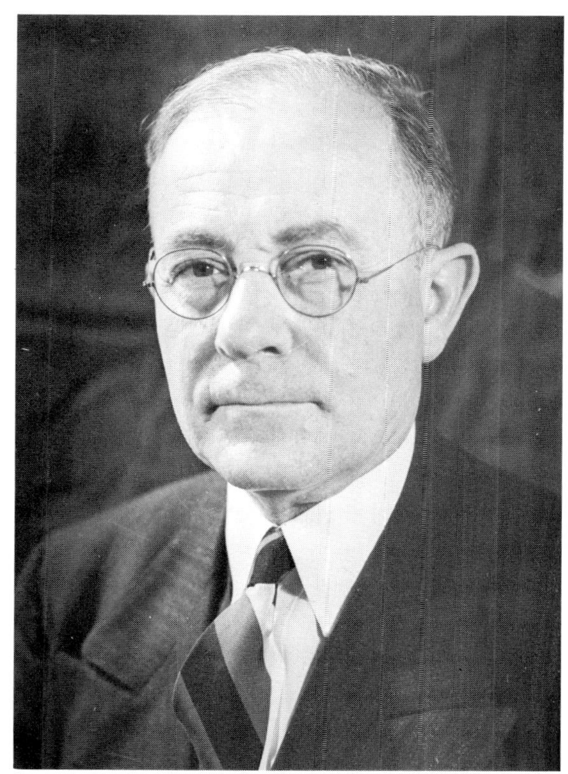

Robert Emmett Burns, 1895–

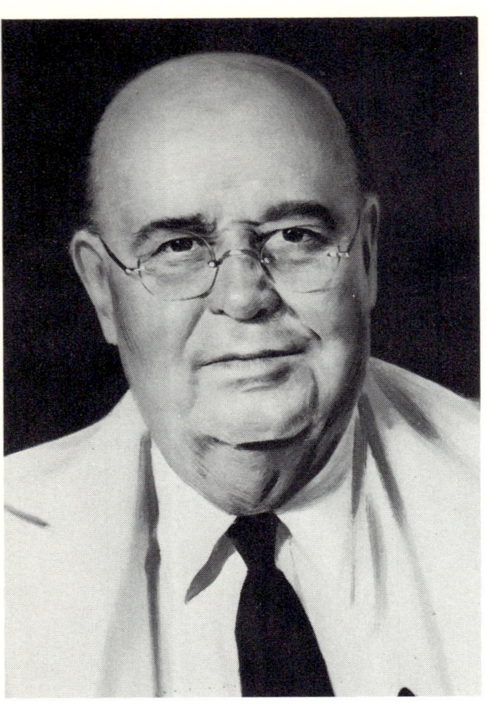

John Warton Harris, 1891–1955.
Portrait by Lester Bentley.

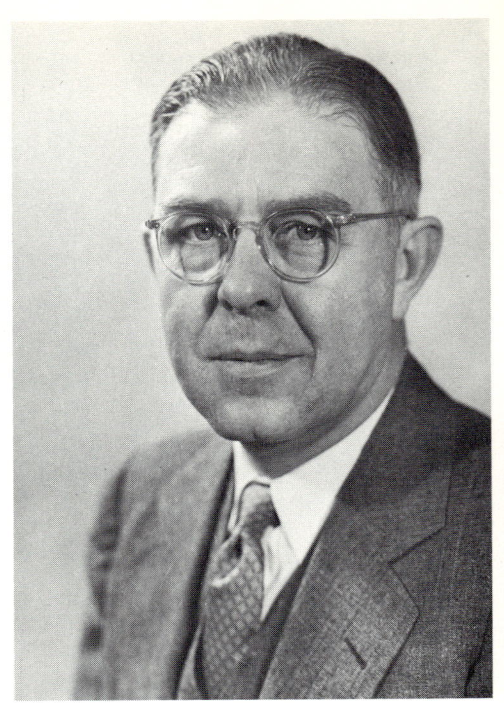

Joseph Wasson Gale, 1900–

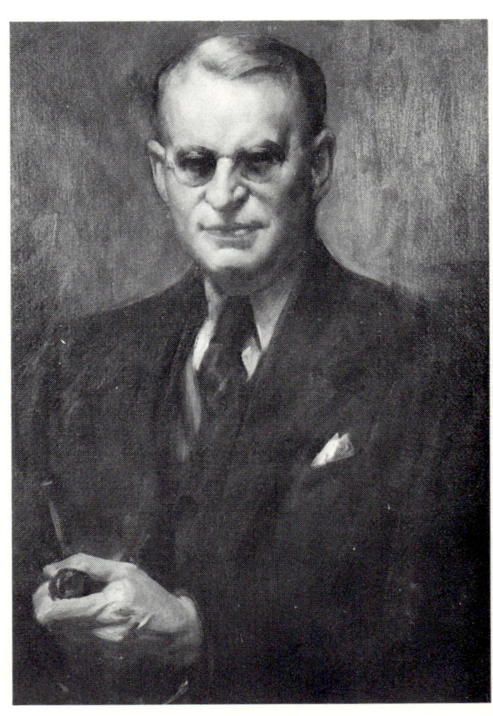

Erwin Rudolph Schmidt, 1890–1961.
Portrait by Myron Nutting.

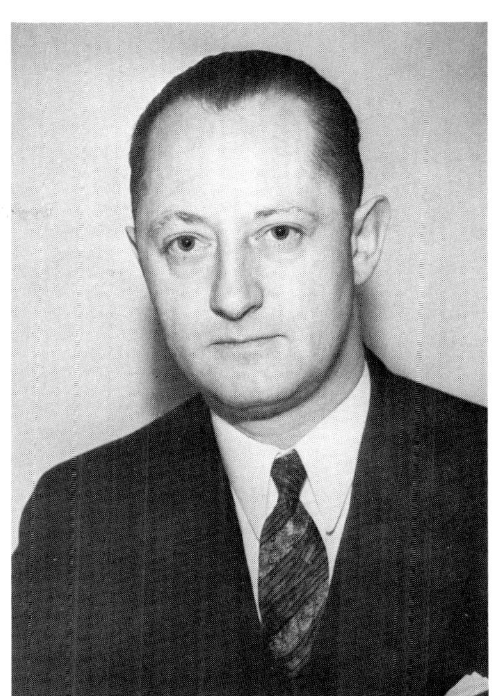

Ernst Albert Pohle,
1885–1965

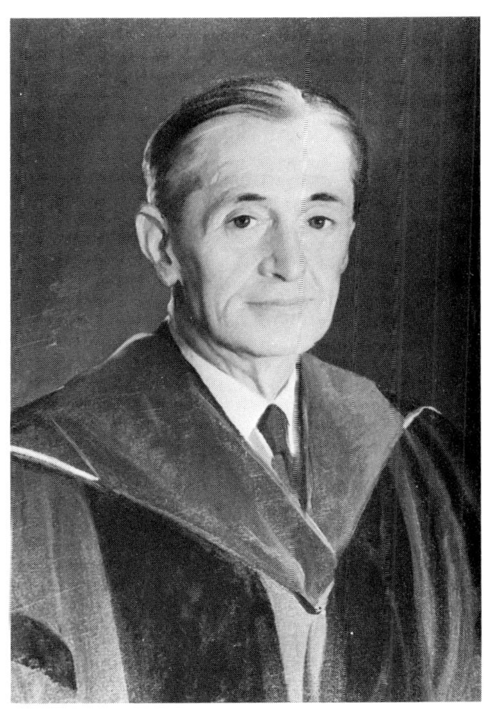

Robert Van Valzah. 1882–1946.
Portrait by B. Eycli.

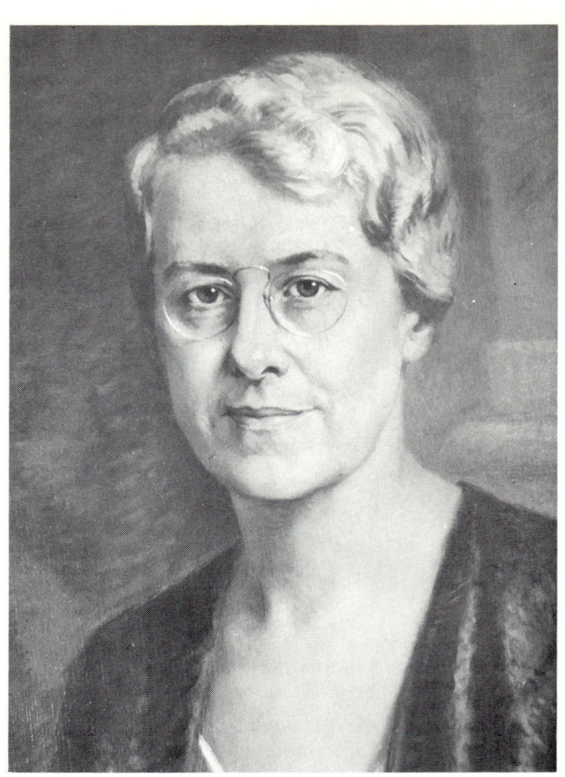

Helen Denne Schulte, 1889–.
Portrait by Herton Grenhagen.

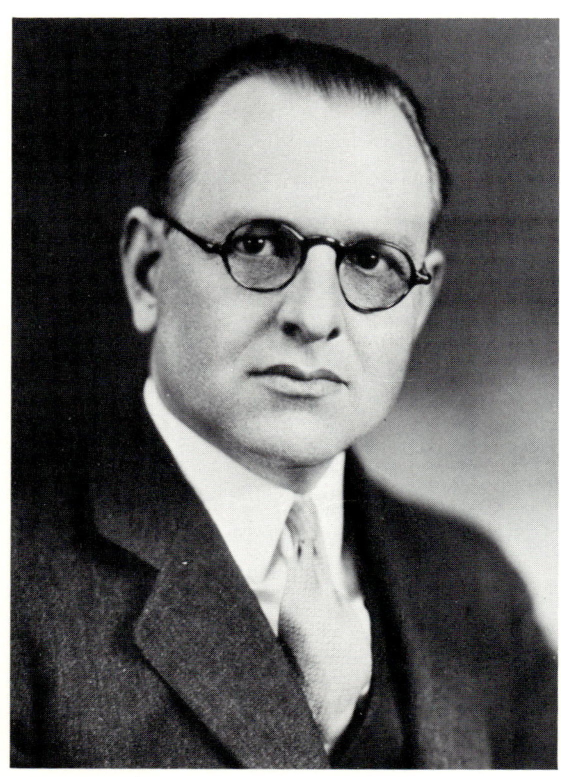

Robin Carl Buerki,
1892–

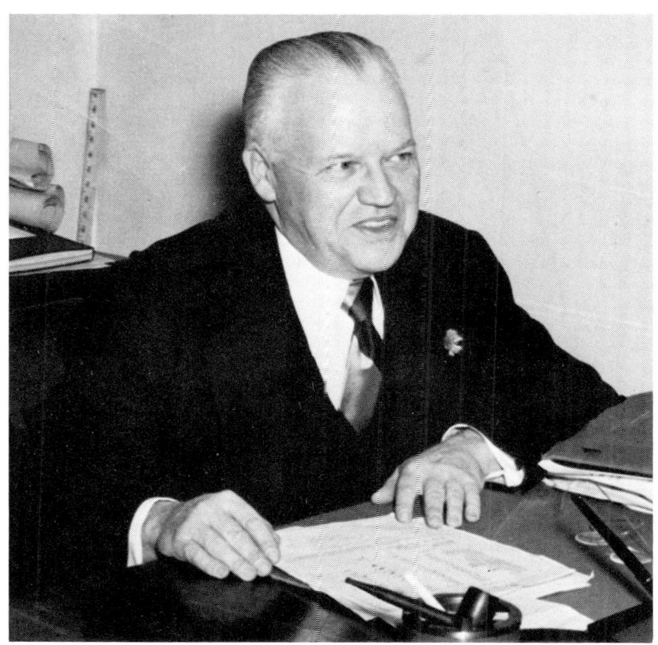

Harold Macomber Coon, 1895–1962

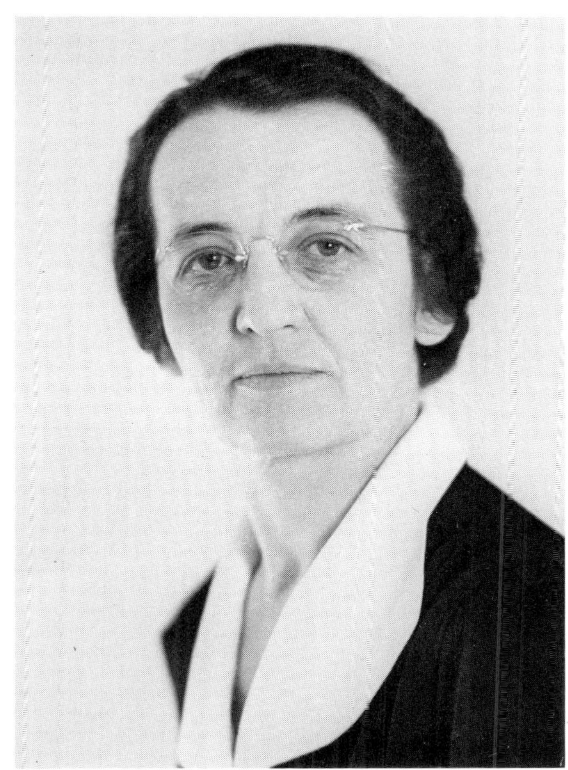

Christina C. Murray,
1896–1948

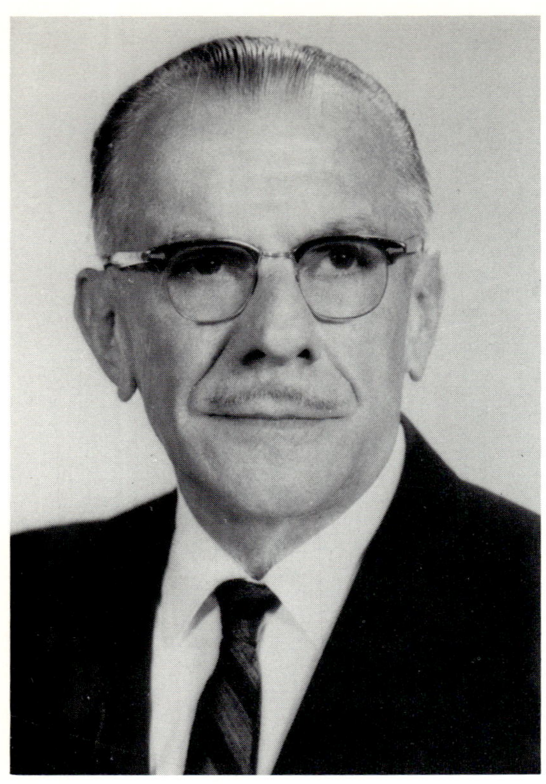

William Jefferson Bleckwenn,
1895–1965

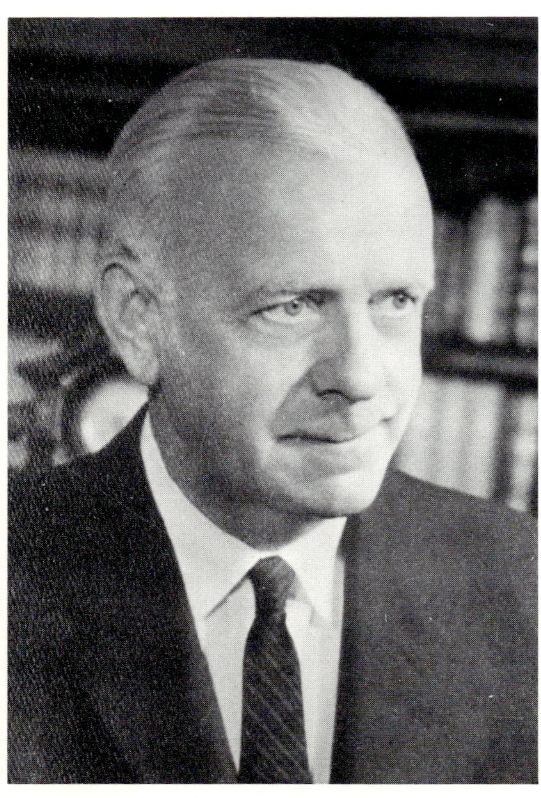

Hans Heinrich Reese, 1891–

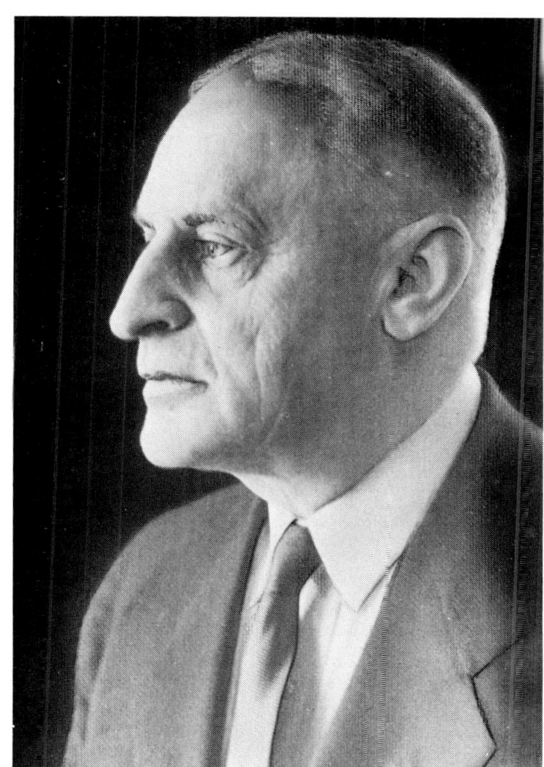

William Frederick Lorenz, 1882–1958

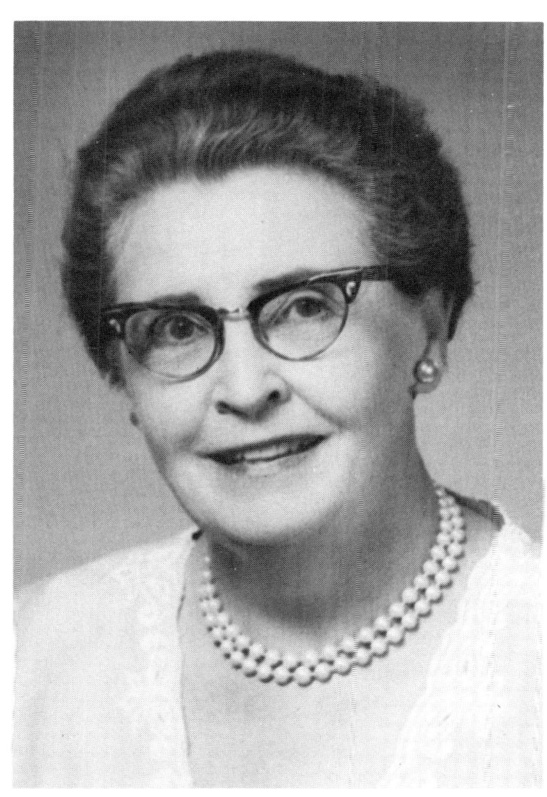

Mabel G. Masten,
1897–

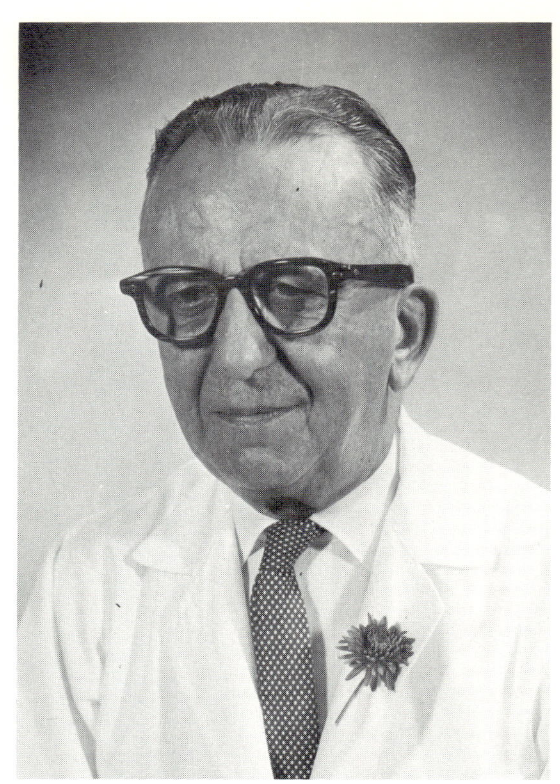

Ovid Otto Meyer,
1900–

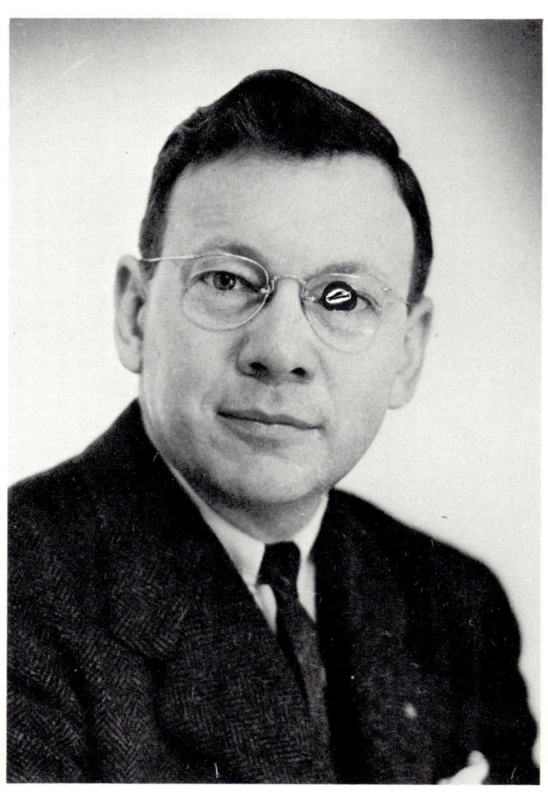

Elmer Louis Sevringhaus,
1894–

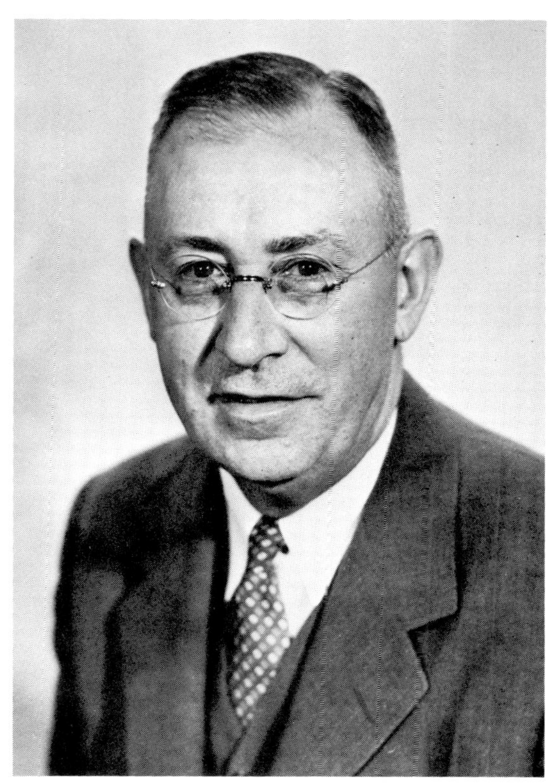

John Eugene Gonce,
1893–1956

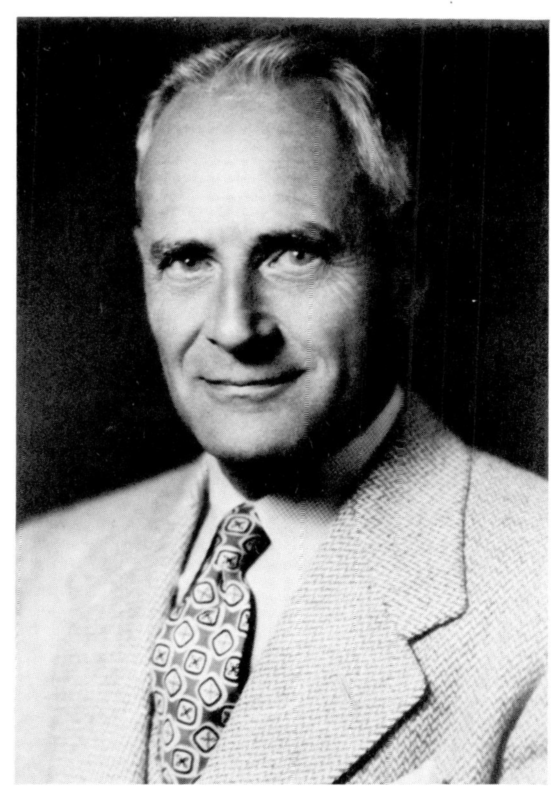

Horace Kent Tenney, Jr.,
1892–

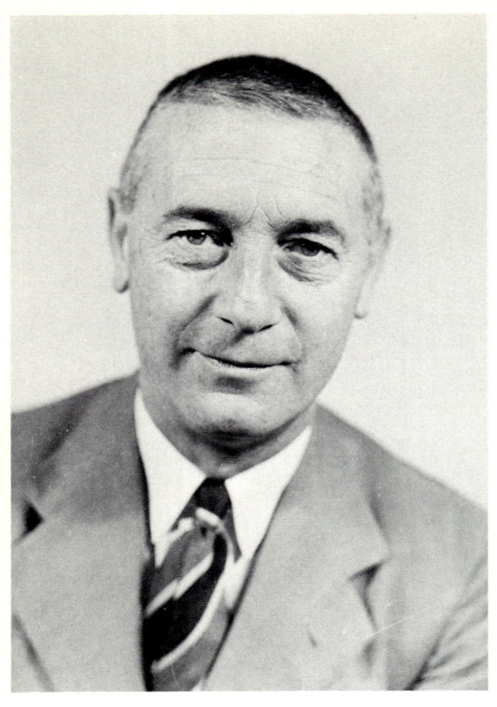

Noel Alexander Gillespie, 1904–1955

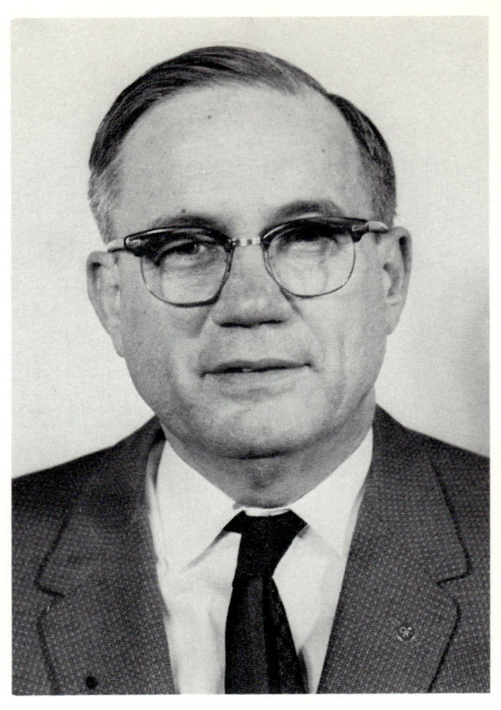

Oswald Sidney Orth, 1906–1964

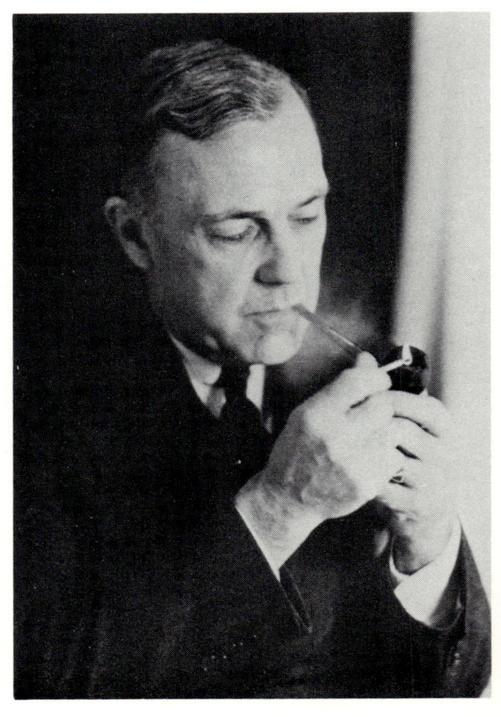

Ralph Milton Waters, 1883–

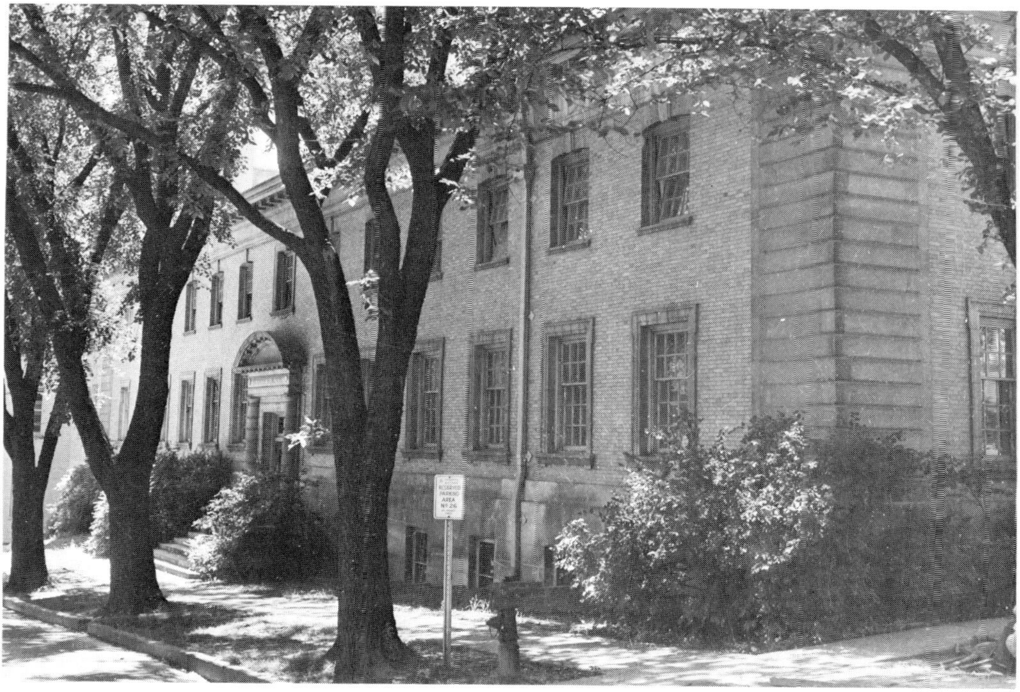

Bradley Memorial Hospital

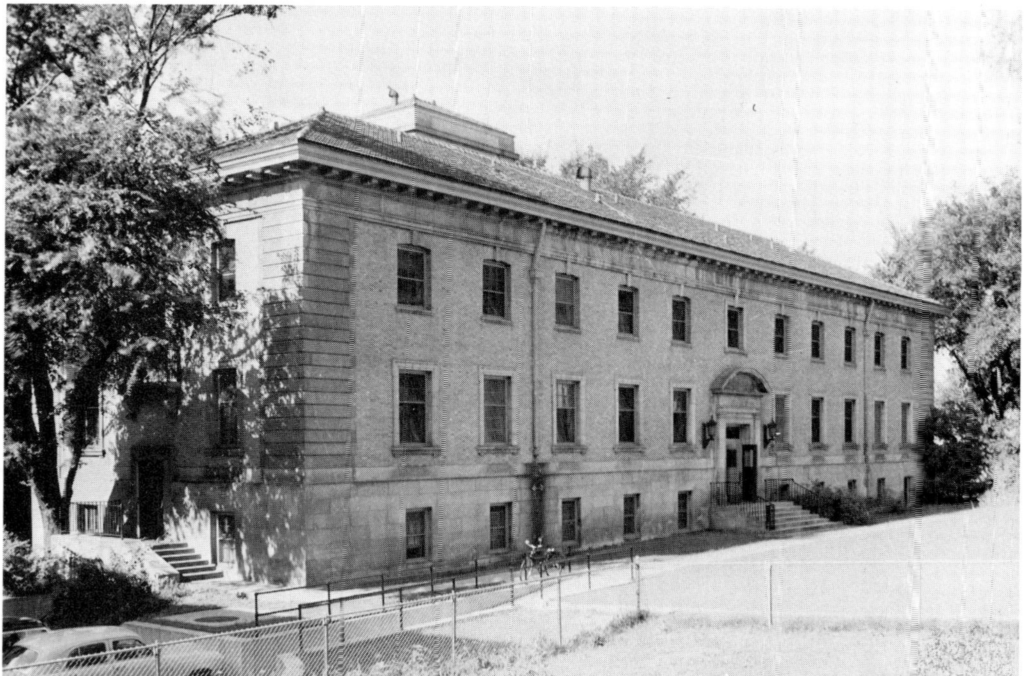

Student Infirmary

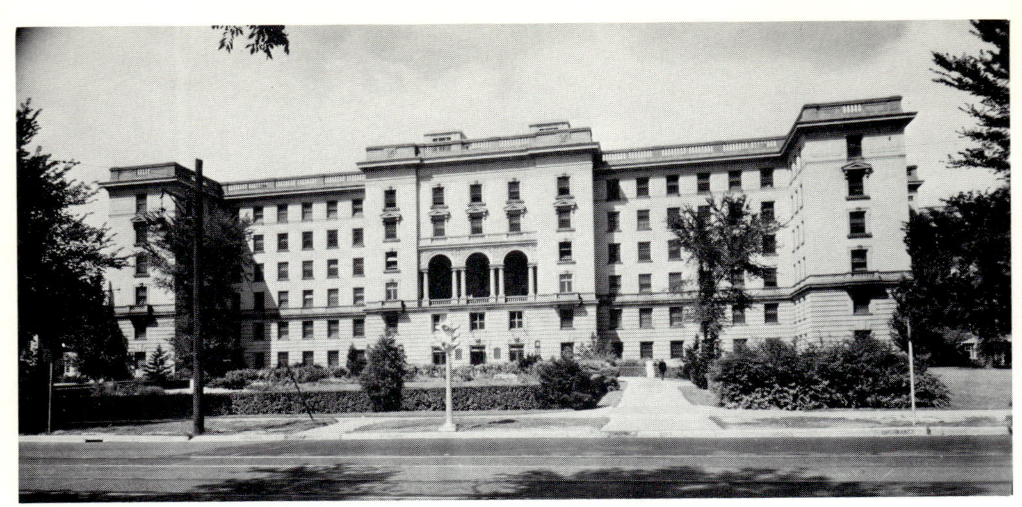

Wisconsin General Hospital, 1925

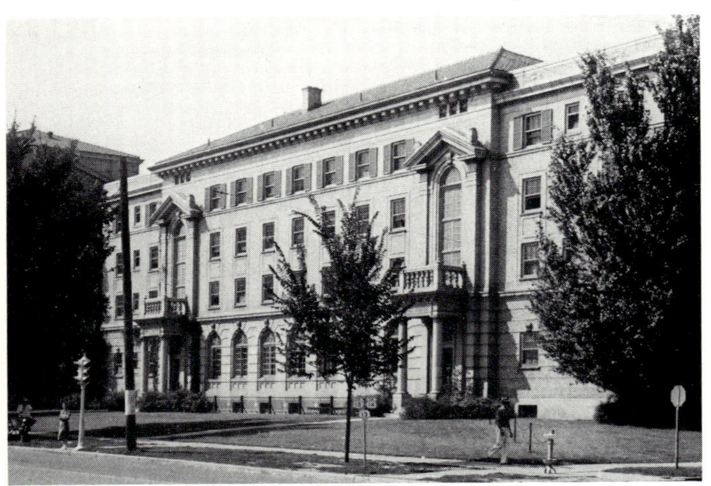

Nurses' Dormitory

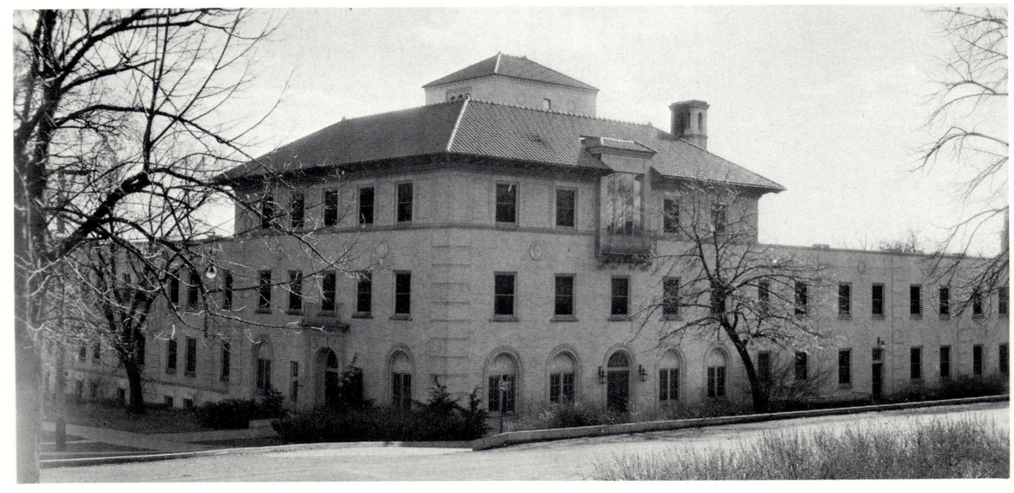

Orthopedic Hospital, *now* Children's Hospital

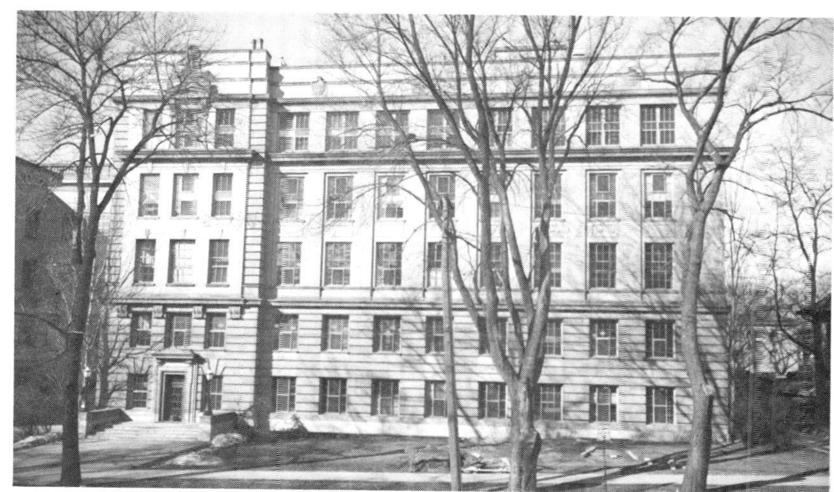

Service Memorial Institutes

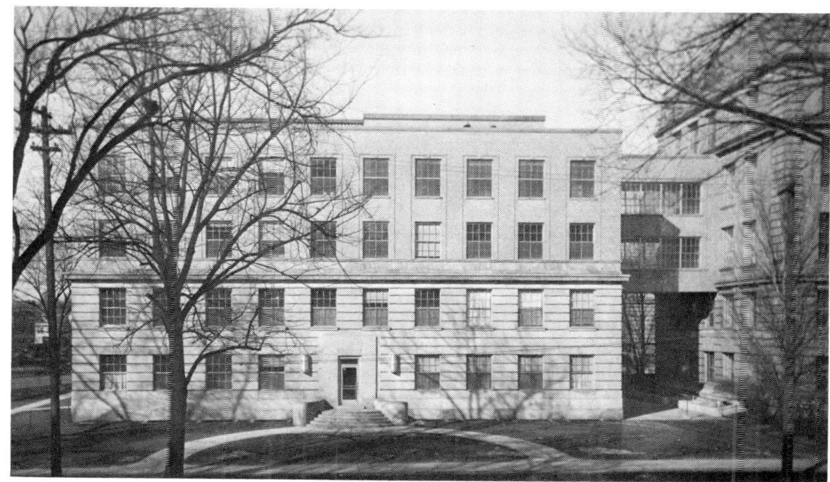

McArdle Laboratory, 1942

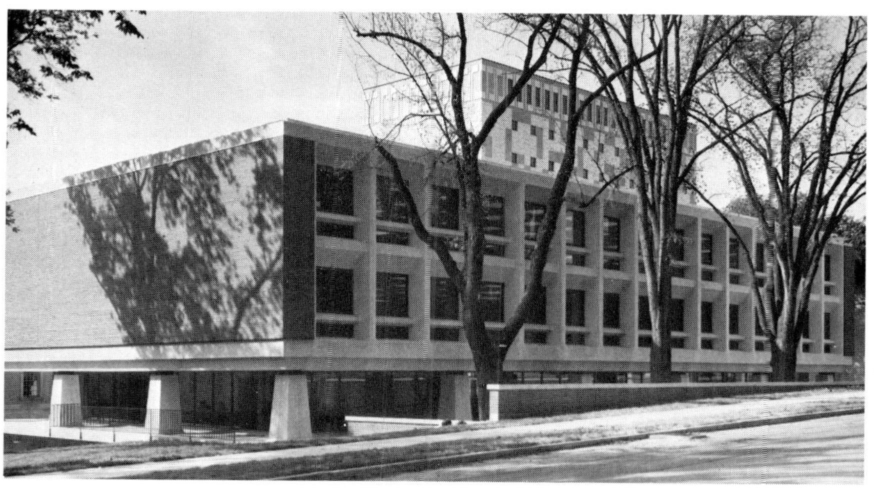

Medical Library

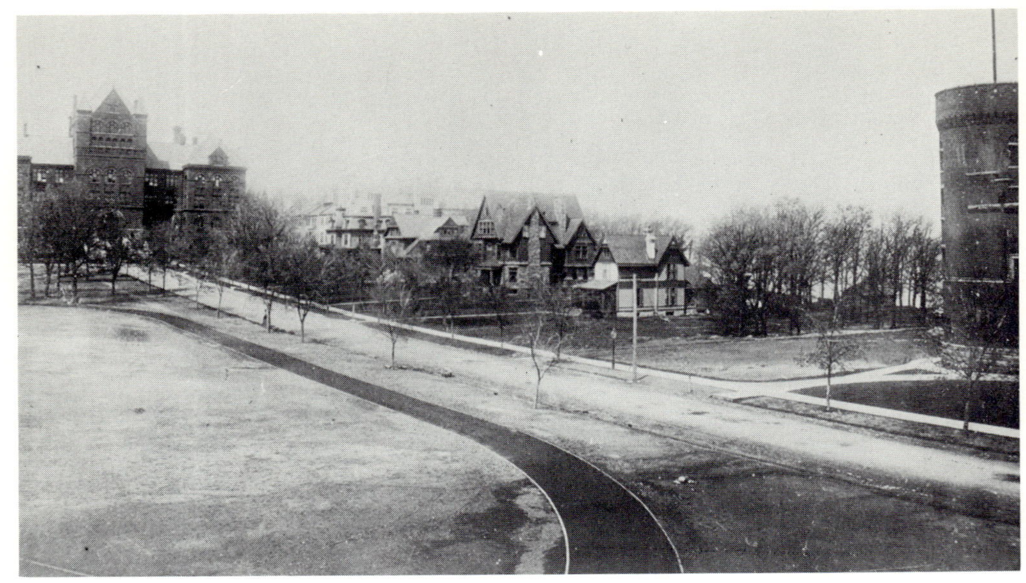

Science Hall and Lower Campus about 1904

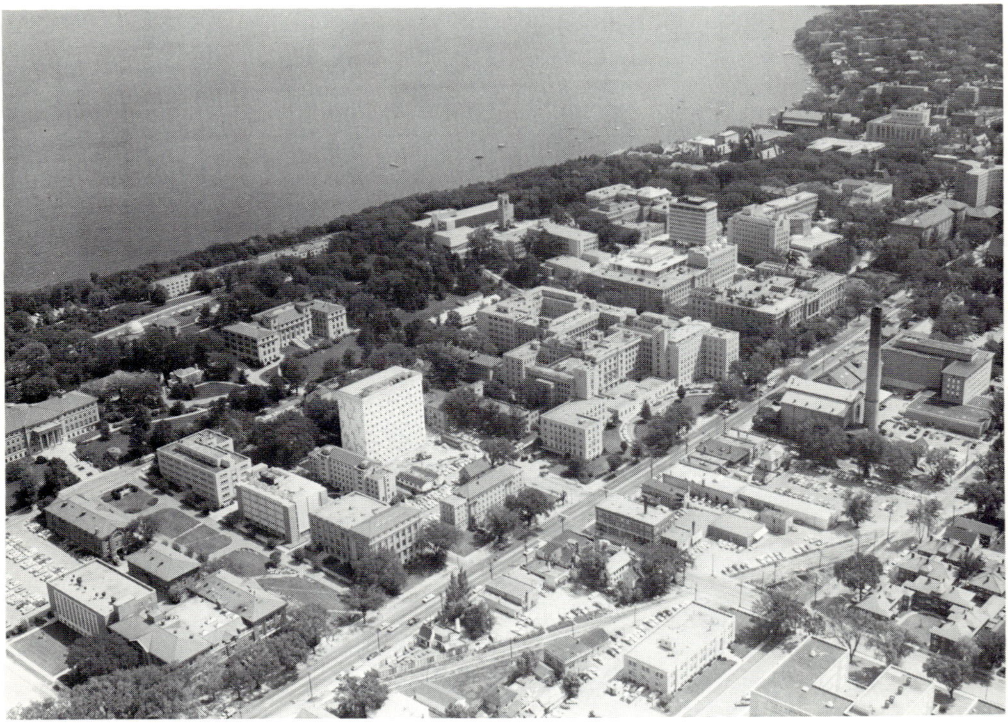

Aerial View of Medical Center, 1965

He did so enjoy planning for the welfare of children, as in the Madison Kiddie Camp, to which he devoted many hours in selecting those children who most needed a few weeks of summer outing with good food and in screening out those who might bring serious infections into the group of vacationers. Later came the convalescent hospital for children with rheumatic fever to provide the required care and discipline rarely obtainable in the home, but so essential for the long convalescence necessary to avoid a lifetime of handicaps. His published contributions, about twenty, came from studies in the home, at the bedside, and from the laboratory — an especially happy combination for a pediatrician. We can name only his studies on the action of ultraviolet rays on the bactericidal property of the blood that were carried on for several years and his many studies on infant feeding, especially the use of citric acid milk.[22]

John — or Slim, as he was affectionately known to his friends — rode several hobbies, but none to excess. Fishing, in Wisconsin and in Florida, golf, gardening, and picnicking kept him in good trim during much of the year. A large and growing collection of stamps, together with his devotion to friends and family, gave him a breadth of interests around the fireside in the winter months. He died in harness as he would have wished. He has been deeply missed both here in the University and in the city.

Dr. Horace Kent Tenney, Jr., has for many years been an integral part of pediatrics here in our Medical School and a much admired physician who has "raised a lot of children here in Madison." His placid assurance and engaging manner with his families has quieted the fears of many a mother and tickled the "funny bone" of the children. He has lived and practiced when pneumonia was "a friend of the aged, and an enemy of the young," and when middle ear infections and scarlet fever were rampant. He has practiced effectively also in these later years when virus diseases have become a byword in our families and both before and after the use of effective vaccination against such devastating childhood diseases as diphtheria, whooping cough, and poliomyelitis. His informal book *Let's Talk About Your Baby* is full of good sense, good medicine, and folksy quips, such as this, from one of the babies, "Vegebles? So that's what it is? Something new to eat." [23] This book should not be allowed to go out of print. It has helped many young mothers and their growing infants. Quite early in his practice, Dr. Tenney realized the importance of behavior problems in children and his article on this subject shows wisdom. Quoting one sentence, "As a matter of fact, if we stated the situation accurately, we should say that we are considering the parents who annoy their children." [24]

Dr. Tenney was born in Chicago, May 11, 1892, and earned his medical degree at Northwestern University Medical School in 1919. He came here as instructor in clinical medicine in the spring of 1920. Officially, he has been on the so-called part-time basis, but that has not kept him from being vitally important in teaching the students throughout his forty-two active years on our staff. Dr. Tenney has traveled widely through the state on medical education programs; his "March of Medicine" radio programs for the State Medical Society have been full of information and insight into human and medical problems. He is at heart and in practice a family doctor.

Recently, Dr. Tenney has expressed "a little fear that with the terrific scientific explosion, we may begin to lose sight of the fact that people are still sick with the same things." He hopes that "the student will not be too concerned with what drugs and techniques to use and forget the individual."

Dr. Tenney has for years been an avid golfer, and earlier he played a fast game of tennis, and was a splendid figure skater. Later he fell a victim to the great sport of skiing; Colorado and other western areas have appreciated his presence and he has enjoyed their chairlifts and slaloms.

Another of our superior pediatricians is Kenneth B. McDonough, a graduate of our University (B.A., Wisconsin, 1927, and M.D., 1930). He was the second physician to complete his residency in pediatrics here (1933); only Dr. Carroll Roach preceded him (1932). Dr. McDonough continued here with growing capacity, advance in the faculty, and with the warm appreciation of his students, who commend especially his correlations of laboratory studies, physical findings in the patient, and specific treatment. His department associates agree that he is a kindly, patient physician. Dr. Tenney has commented, "In all the years I have known him, I have never heard any expression of exasperation with an individual or a situation. An underlying chuckle is an integral part of every conversation anyone has with him. He has gone through personal and family illness time after time, but it has never 'got him down.' " He worked with Dr. Gonce in the upbuilding of the Kiddie Camp. Of his

published papers, his favorites are, "The treatment of meningitis," and
"A study of the relation of rickets to anemia." [25]

An excellent example of the way the University of Wisconsin uses its
opportunities for intellectual cross-fertilization is found in another member of the pediatrics group. With the Ph.D. degree, earned in 1939 under
Conrad Elvehjem, from the biochemistry department of the College of
Agriculture, Dr. Harry A. Waisman has followed winding paths all leading eventually to an important position in the pediatrics world. By 1941,
Waisman had turned his attention to the influence of diet on resistance
to virus diseases, chiefly experimental infantile paralysis and related diseases of the central nervous system. These studies were carried on in a
specially constructed virus laboratory out in the western part of the campus. Over a number of years, the possible relationship of exactly determined diets in *Macacus rhesus* monkeys and mice to resistance to induced infections was studied by a group with Elvehjem and Waisman
chiefly responsible for the nutrition end and with Clark and Rasmussen
for the virus end of the experiments.[26]

Waisman received the M.D. degree here at Wisconsin in 1947; then
the University of Illinois claimed him in pediatrics. It was not until a
few years after our terminal date that Waisman returned to Wisconsin,
where he has been carrying on capably in the department of pediatrics.
His important contributions coming from this department must necessarily be left for some later historian to present.

RESIDENTS IN PEDIATRICS THROUGH 1950

1932	Carroll E. Roach
1933	Kenneth B. McDonough
1935	Harold Fechtner
	Bessie Shebesta Heald
1939	Eugenia E. Murphy
1941	George E. Oosterhous
1947	James S. Vedder
1948	John R. Paul, Jr.
1949	Melvin G. Apell
1950	Jean S. LePoidevin
	Patricia E. McIllece
	Edward Zupanc

PULMONARY DISEASE

The first member of the department of medicine who specialized in pulmonary diseases was Dr. Reuben H. Stiehm; he was born in 1901 at Johnson Creek, Wisconsin, and died in Madison at the age of forty on October 21, 1941. After his early schooling, he spent one year here at the University and then transferred to the University of Indiana, where he earned his medical degree in 1926; he served an internship and also a medical residency at Wisconsin General Hospital. Following a brief period in private practice, he accepted a position with the Wisconsin Anti-Tuberculosis Association. That experience set the pattern of his professional life. In 1933 he joined the Student Health Service of the University; pulmonary disease, especially tuberculosis, became his continuing, absorbing interest. He began a never-ending and rewarding search for pre-symptomatic cases of tuberculosis, with a tuberculin testing program among the students and repeated gastric aspirations in the search for tubercle bacilli. He realized that tuberculosis could be eliminated as a health hazard chiefly through the discovery of these early cases that were occasionally shedding the bacilli.[27]

One of the more significant of Dr. Stiehm's studies was that concerned with the comparison of intracutaneous reactions to the purified protein derivative of several species of acid-fast bacilli. This was carried out with Drs. Janet McCarter and Horace Getz, a good example of interdepartmental collaboration.[28] Their suggestion that some of the reactors may have been sensitized by other mycobacteria commonly considered non-pathogenic has been proved true in studies by later investigators; these organisms have been shown to have some pathogenic properties for man with dosage as a considerable factor.

Dr. Stiehm had a warm, quietly gay attitude toward his patients, especially the children he cared for in his work at Morningside Sanatorium. He was much appreciated both by his patients and by members of the medical profession. All mourned his deplorably early death.

Many have been involved here at Wisconsin in the anti-tuberculosis campaign. We are immediately reminded of the startling results and the importance of Dean Russell's application of the tuberculin test in the University herd of cattle back in 1894. Dr. Stiehm's yearly tuberculin skin test survey of the University of Wisconsin students with X-rays of the reactors brought to light seventy-one cases of active tuberculosis within five years.

Dr. William A. Oatway, Jr., in 1936, conducted one of the nation's early studies of tuberculosis in general hospitals and found 2.3 per cent of admissions to the Wisconsin General Hospital had active tuberculosis. He stressed the importance of routine chest X-raying of patients admitted to general hospitals. He and Dr. Middleton developed the attractive seventh-floor air-conditioned isolation unit for all suspected cases of tuberculosis.[29]

Dr. Oatway could properly be pictured under several phases of his interesting life. He took his B.S. degree at Wisconsin in 1924, including his first two years of medical training; he was so good in pathology that Dr. Bunting invited him to stay on the following year as instructor in the course. He completed the work for the M.D. degree at the University of Pennsylvania in 1928. For the next few years he acquired broadening medical experience in a variety of positions, as a resident and instructor in medicine at Wisconsin from 1929 to 1931 and professional appointments at the Trudeau and other sanatoria and at the Thorndike Laboratories at Harvard through 1935. He returned to Wisconsin, earning appreciation and advancement until he left for war work in 1942. Dr. Oatway published a number of significant studies in tuberculosis of which we may cite one on hematology and another on broad biological studies on the tubercle bacilli with Steenken and Petroff.[30]

Dr. Oatway was outgoing and easy to know so that both students and older colleagues enjoyed being with him. To our regret, he did not return to Wisconsin after the war but found congenial professional opportunity in a milder climate. He was devoted also to several of the fine arts; his portrait bronze of Dr. Evans, whom he knew intimately, is splendid. It tells us more of "the chief" than the painted portraits by professional artists.

Of the several attempts at the history of the Medical School, Oatway's history of the school, 1880–1923, written for the Miller history seminar in 1939 is the most personal; it includes a volume of selected photographs of the early faculty and buildings.[31] I wish that he might have been my collaborator in these efforts.

After Dr. Oatway had left Wisconsin (he became the director of the La Viña Sanatorium, Altadena, California), Dr. Helen Dickie became our responsible leader in the anti-tuberculosis studies. With the concerted campaign against tuberculosis throughout the country and the world, the incidence of the disease among University of Wisconsin students has diminished, but routine search has shown five to ten new cases yearly. The search continues.

Dr. Helen A. Dickie, a native of Wisconsin, took both her letters and science work here in the University and also that for the medical degree, which she obtained in 1937. Several years spent at the Los Angeles County Hospital as an intern and then as a resident in tuberculosis gave her the basis for her subsequent deep interest in pulmonary disease. She returned to Wisconsin and was appointed in preventive medicine and student health in 1941–42. She has continued to advance in experience and in rank, attaining at the end of our historical period the rank of associate professor and renown as a specialist in tuberculosis. We may cite her important studies on spontaneous mediastinal emphysema and spontaneous pneumothorax.[32] She is admired for her forthright statements, her clinical acumen, especially in difficult chest cases, her productive work, and her down-to-earth positions on moot subjects.

In presenting this brief account of the study and treatment of pulmonary disease in the Medical School, it would be a gross omission if we failed to mention the annual Dearholt Day in honor of Dr. Hoyt E. Dearholt, so long the Wisconsin leader against the "Captain of the Men of Death." Each year the message is repeated by important investigators who continue the struggle to drive the tuberculosis figures, both morbidity and mortality, to lower and lower levels.

GENERAL MEDICINE

By the time of my terminal dates of 1948–50, many of the competent younger physicians in the large, developing department of medicine were becoming dependable, productive men in the middle-aged group. By the time this history appears between brilliant cardinal covers, some who were my students will have climbed all the way to the top of their profession, some will have joined the emeritus group, and some, to my sorrow, will have passed beyond that point.

The younger, active members of this and other departments must, to a large degree, be left to the tender mercies of some future historian. All I can do is to give them warm appreciation and best wishes. We delight in them; they provide us with high expectations. The reader will

understand, I am sure, that my sketches of persons living at the time of
the writing must be thought of more as chronicles rather than objective
critical history.

Dr. Frank L. Weston took his undergraduate studies and his first two
years of medical training here at the University of Wisconsin, completing
the work for the M.D. degree at Rush Medical College, 1923, with subsequent internships at Cook County and Presbyterian Hospitals, Chicago.
While a student here, he was an outstanding athlete, captain of the football team during his senior year, and a fine basketball player. Save for
leave of absence for military service 1942–45, Dr. Weston has continued
here from 1925 to a time far beyond our terminal date.

Weston is a shining example of a devoted medical practitioner, loved
and trusted by his patients, who, while on a so-called part-time basis, has
contributed abundantly to the care of patients in the hospital and to vivid
analytical teaching of the students. He has a remarkable talent for interweaving his many tasks and patients. He loves medical practice; those
associated with him in whatever capacity deeply appreciate the relationship. With Dr. Karver Puestow, he has for years had charge of outpatients, a growing and essential service in the hospital both for treatment
and for teaching. Such dedicated practicing physicians on our faculty
make the policy of exclusively using full-time appointments as carried
out in several well-endowed private medical schools seem less important
and even undesirable. The man in competitive practice has much to offer
to the student who is himself going out into competitive practice.

Dr. Weston's professional interests are in all phases of general medicine, and the number of patients both in and out of the hospital who de-
pend on his splendid skill and care is astounding. Dr. Weston has published very few papers; he has been too busy caring for the sick.

Ball games with the children and grandchildren, an occasional wield-
ing of the tennis racket, and moderately vigorous daily exercises have
replaced the football field, save when he is an enthusiastic spectator.
However, he tackles all problems with his accustomed zeal.

Dr. Marie Louise Carns obtained her several degrees and much of her
training at the University of Wisconsin; she received her M.D. degree
with our first graduating class in 1927. Always precise and effective,
she continued her active advancement in the department of medicine until

1946 when she became professor and director of the physical education department for women. We remember with pleasure her sharp succinct remarks at the clinical pathological conferences. She left no doubt where she stood in the matter of a difficult differential diagnosis. One of her favorite papers was written with her long-time close associate, Dr. Annette C. Washburne, on "Psychiatric investigation in internal medicine." [33]

Frederick John Pohle, 1906–47, a native of Wisconsin, received his doctor of medicine degree from the University of Michigan in 1934; while in medical school, he assisted in hematologic research at the Simpson Memorial Institute. After serving both an internship and a residency in medicine at Wisconsin General Hospital, he became a research fellow at Harvard Medical School and assistant physician at the Thorndike Memorial Laboratory and Boston City Hospital. He returned to the University of Wisconsin in 1938 to become a research associate and later an assistant professor of medicine. After distinguished service in World War II, he returned to the University of Wisconsin and was associate professor of medicine at the time of his death, November 26, 1947.

Dr. Pohle had an innate sympathy and appreciation of his associates whether patient, student, or colleague. His major research interest was hematology, a field to which he made significant contributions.[34] His enthusiasm for his research projects, his skill as a physician, and his consideration for others made his untimely death deeply felt by all his colleagues.

Dr. John LeRoy Sims, a native Texan and a graduate of Rice Institute in 1933 and the University of Texas Medical School in 1937, came here as an intern in 1937. His excellence in teaching, care of patients, and investigation kept him here through residency in internal medicine and had carried him to an assistant professorship by our terminal date; a prophet is not needed to predict further merited advance. His field of special interest is diseases of the liver.[35]

RESIDENTS IN MEDICINE THROUGH 1950

1926	Mark J. Bach
1928	Edwin McKinley
1929	Ovid O. Meyer

1930	Gerald W. Shaw
	Reuben H. Stiehm
1931	Nels A. Hill
	William H. Oatway
1933	Adolph Hutter
	Paul H. Schmiedicke
	Calvin M. Yoran
1934	Sam Boyer
	Horace R. Getz
	Howard J. Lee
	Harold P. Rusch
	John A. Stiles
1935	Scott Goodnight, Jr.
	C. F. Midelfart
	Alexander T. Ross
	William C. Sheehan
1936	Einar Daniels
	Edgar S. Gordon
	Frederick J. Pohle
1937	F. S. Robinson
	H. H. Shapiro
1938	Ben J. Axel
	Winifred Ingersoll
	Walter H. Jaeschke
	Reno R. Porter
1939	Robin N. Allin
	James O. Burke
	Eleanor Cheydleur
	Bernice L. Eversmeyer
	Meyer Friedman
	Thoralf Gundersen
	Hugh A. Kennedy
	Jackman Pyre
1940	S. R. Edwards
	William M. Faber
	Norton E. Humphrey
	C. Selby Mills
	Herbert W. Pohle

1941	James B. Bingham
	Stephan W. Brouwer
	Julian R. Kaufman
	Roy B. Larson
	William E. Leede
	Arthur S. Tucker
	Isabel J. Wolfstein
1942	John L. Bell
	Dante Castrodale
	Helen P. Davis
	Richard R. Davis
	Helen Dickie
	Dan S. Ellis
	Francis C. Johnson
	Ralph R. Meyer
	J. L. Sims
1943	Joseph H. Batzle
	Octavio Germek
	Donald O. Prasser
	Ruth St. John
	Jerome Sugarman
	Charles J. Thill
1944	Margaret N. Bingham
	Gabriel Fournier
	Roland F. Knox
	Helen S. Marshall
	Ulises G. Martinez
	Rolf F. Poser
	Renato Sanz
	Gonzalo Sepulveda
	James M. Wilkie
1945	Richard D. Moore
	Stella H. Sikkema
1946	Herbert Shulman
	Frank W. VanKirk, Jr.
1947	Francis E. Gehin
	Elizabeth Grimm
1948	Edwin C. Albright

          Jack E. Clifford
          Ephraim B. Cohen
          Charles W. Crumpton
          John J. Halbert
          William E. Jones
          John T. McCoy
          Paul J. Reinsch
          Robert F. Schilling
          John G. Verberkmoes
          Arvin B. Weinstein
          Harold C. Youngreen
1949   Robert W. Ramlow
          Anthony J. Richtsmeier
          Harold J. Tausend
1950   William D. Battle
          Dean B. Becker, Jr.
          Frank C. Larson
          Thomas H. Lorenz
          Marie B. Webster

20 The Medical Library and the
Department of the History of Medicine

For books are not absolutely dead things, but do contain a potency of life in them to be as active as that soul was whose progeny they are; nay, they do preserve as in a vial the purest efficacy and extraction of that living intellect that bred them.

John Milton

Money invested in a library gives much better return than mining stock.

William Osler

Files of the more important journals as well as substantial texts in the underlying sciences on which medicine is based were in the University libraries before the Medical School was more than a dream in the minds of Van Hise, Birge, and a few others.[1] Dr. Bardeen's appointment as professor of anatomy (1904) and Erlanger's as professor of physiology (1906) were indicative of the future, and each of them began to use available library funds to order important journals in their respective fields. Bardeen also made available a few journals and some of his personal library in his office in the Olin house on Langdon Street where the Union now stands. The completeness and range of the journal sets is now one of the great strengths of the library.

When the northwest wing of the State Historical Library was completed in 1914, the University was permitted to use these facilities; the Medical School Library shared the space with other departments. In 1924 a room on the fourth floor of the north wing of the newly constructed hospital became our first separate medical library; here, files and current numbers of the most-used journals and important texts were shelved. When the Service Memorial Institutes were planned in 1926–27,

156

space was attractively designed for the medical library.[2] Because of lack of room in the hospital for Dr. Pohle and the new department of radiology, this library space next to the hospital was surrendered to that need, and space that had been planned for the dean's offices and the machine shop near Charter Street was given over to library use.

At the Charter Street entrance of the Institutes building, paintings by Professor Roland Stebbins and his assistants and a colorful stained glass window with the Aesculapian staff in the center provided an appropriate memorial foyer. Exhibit cases in the center of the room gave opportunity for a series of monthly exhibits arranged for many years by Mrs. Paul F. Clark, a former medical librarian, to show events and persons of medical historical interest.[3] In later years, the department of the history of medicine and the growing library were compelled by the need for space to take over most of this attractive entrance room, leaving just enough space for passageway. A serious hazard in a basement stock room has been the threat of floods; one of these caused irreparable damage to a section of the bound journals through the bursting of overhead hot water pipes. Despite the inadequate physical facilities, the medical library has grown in strength and effectiveness.

Through all the years our library staff has consisted of an enthusiastic group of librarians, all of them eager to be of service to students and faculty. Miss Frances Van Zandt was our first graduate librarian from 1927 to 1931. She was followed by Miss Gladys Ramsey from 1931 to 1944, and then by Miss Helen Crawford in 1946, who was the first academic appointee. Named associate professor in 1949, Miss Crawford has been highly capable in reference aid and book selection, and of inestimable value during our period of rapid growth and planning for the future. The medical library committee, especially their several chairmen, beginning with Dr. Miller, have through the decades served useful functions both in the selection of books and journals and in the rejection of some over-enthusiastic requests. While we were still a small family, Mrs. Minnie Loevenhart, widow of Dr. Arthur Loevenhart, was for years (1931–46) gracious but firm at the delivery desk, and Miss Celia Harriman (later Mrs. Arthur Tatum) rendered excellent support in the Medical Library Service.

Purchases and acquisitions have in the past been financed mainly through University Library funds, with occasional welcome gifts. Personnel and other costs are borne by the Medical School budget. In addition to the vitally important and continuing sets of journals, our medical history collection contains many treasures. The initial gift of Drs. Byron Robinson and Lucy Waite in 1910 included works by authors such as Albinus, Chelselden, Hewson, Charles Bell, Cooper, Bartlett, and Eberle. Another generous contributor was Dr. Maurice L. Richardson, who had been a member of the first William Snow Miller medical history seminar and had retained his interest in rare books and in medical history. Among his valuable gifts were the Latin translation of the Moslem physician Avenzoar (1497) and Hooke's *Micrographia*. Other gifts include a rare 1530 edition of Hippocrates from Dr. Merritt Jones, a first edition of Dr. William Beaumont's *Experiments and Observations on the Gastric Juice* from George Haight, a generous University benefactor, and volumes by Boerhaave, Abercrombie, Skoda, Mueller, and Sydenham given by Dr. J. A. E. Eyster after his retirement. The library is indebted to many physicians and their heirs for individual items of interest and value.[4]

The most extensive single collection is the William Snow Miller library, which was purchased by the Regents for $15,000 after the death of Dr. Miller in 1940. It is particularly strong in text books of anatomy and the history of medicine, including the first (1543) and second (1545) Basel editions of the *Fabrica* by Vesalius.[5]

In addition to meeting the needs here in Madison, the library has provided bibliographic aid to physicians throughout the state. In 1927, the Medical School, the Extension Division, and the State Medical Society cooperated to inaugurate this service which is now supported entirely by the Medical School. Books, periodicals, and reference service are made available to physicians, clinics, and citizens of the state. Nearly one-third of the state's population live in areas where there is no organized library service, and although a larger proportion of doctors are located in cities, many of the individual borrowers from the Medical Library Service have no local library well enough staffed to process inter-library loan requests.[6]

In 1946, Mr. Thomas Brittingham, frequent benefactor of the University, told Dean Middleton that he would provide funds to establish a medical school professorship not supported by the regular University budget. This offer eventually brought to our campus, in 1947, Dr. Erwin H. Ackerknecht (M.D., University of Leipzig) as our first professor of the history of medicine. With his ardent personality, his flair for vivid speech, and his detailed scholarship, he made an unusual place for himself on our campus and as an international scholar. His interest in the French clinical school has given the library a superior collection of the French authors of the late eighteenth and early nineteenth centuries.

Early in his service as dean, Dr. Middleton set aside a small money gift from an alumnus who wished to express his gratitude to the Medical School in a tangible manner. Later, the Dean suggested a long-range plan, the establishment of a special alumni fund for the construction of a beautiful and adequate medical library. Stirred by this vision, some of the far-seeing alumni began to promote this idea. Although both the two- and the four-year alumni have always been loyal and active, a specific plan, like the Middleton Medical Library, was necessary to focus their efforts. The Wisconsin Medical Alumni, under the unflagging, courageous leadership of Mischa Lustok (M.D., Wisconsin, 1935), have done the "impossible." They have collected well over half a million dollars to construct a beautiful, commodious library to honor their distinguished teacher of medicine, Dr. William S. Middleton.

21   Department of Surgery

Joy, temperance and repose
slam the door on the doctor's nose.
Code of Health, Salerno, Twelfth Century

Until 1920 when the Bradley Memorial Hospital and the Student Infirmary were completed, the major surgical needs of the students were met by Madison physicians or by those in the home areas of the students. The first regular surgical services established in the Medical School were those of plastic surgery with Dr. G. V. I. Brown in charge and orthopedic surgery in the hands of Dr. Frederick J. Gaenslen. Just as the Student Health Service was the bridge to the development of the department of medicine for the third and fourth years of the Medical School, so these surgical specialties, especially orthopedic surgery, provided the early pathway for the department of surgery.

ORTHOPEDIC SURGERY

Dr. Frederick Julius Gaenslen (1877–1937) was born in Milwaukee of German parents. With his undergraduate work at the University of Wisconsin (B.S., 1899), his medical degree at Johns Hopkins (1903), three years at the German Hospital in New York, and repeated visits to active clinics in this country and in Europe, he had had an excellent education. From 1912, he restricted his practice to orthopedic surgery and became a recognized leader with professorships both at Marquette and the University of Wisconsin medical schools.

In 1920, he was appointed orthopedic surgeon (part-time) in our school and was successful in developing an active service. Dr. Gaenslen was handsome, immaculately groomed, and highly competent both technically and in diagnosis; he acquired a large circle of warm admirers and grateful patients. On his weekly trips to Madison, he used to stay in the old student infirmary on Langdon Street. He would review the cases with his younger associates in the evening and be up bright and early the next morning to start his work at the Bradley Hospital. He operated rapidly, but was meticulous and careful. He was skillful also in the older manipulative procedures. He represented a happy combination of the old and the new both in method and in person. His residents especially enjoyed his warm interest in their development and his attention to detail. His instructions to patients were also detailed and specific.

Throughout his life, Dr. Gaenslen contributed an extensive and varied series of papers, some on new techniques, subsequently widely adopted, others on congenital malformations, and, in broader fields, essays on preventive medicine and physical therapy. We can cite only a few of his publications.[1]

It is a pleasure to remember Dr. Gaenslen and to acknowledge the debt the Medical School and his students owe him. He was so gracious and likeable that even those who had only slight contact with him had a warm feeling toward him. He was a choice spirit. His program for the crippled children of the state still goes on, and in Milwaukee we find the Gaenslen School for these unfortunates. Here in Madison we owe much to him for his aid in obtaining the Orthopedic (now Children's) Hospital. We also owe him a debt of gratitude for training excellent orthopedic surgeons throughout the state and especially the two men, Dr. Robert E. Burns and Dr. Herman W. Wirka, who have earned the warm appreciation of patients and colleagues as his successors.

Dr. Robert E. Burns, a native of Wisconsin, took his undergraduate studies and first two years of medical training here at the University (B.S., 1917) and served also as a part-time assistant in anatomy during 1915–17. He completed his studies for the M.D. degree at the University of Pennsylvania in 1919. Two years, 1919–21, at the Hospital for the Ruptured and Crippled in New York and a fellowship in orthopedic surgery at the Mayo Clinic prepared him for the years of successful growth in his specialty with Dr. Gaenslen. Increasingly, Dr. Burns took over the full-time responsibilities of orthopedic surgery, with appropriate recognitions in rank and a professorship in 1932.

Following the death of Dr. Gaenslen (1937), Dr. Burns became the head of orthopedic surgery, a position he has filled with distinction for many years. Dr. Burns has been a skillful surgeon and has in turn trained others successfully. He believes in training the young surgeon at the operating table. To quote him: "Surgeons are made at the elbow of another surgeon." The smallest detail is never overlooked. His favorite quote is, "Trifles make perfection, but perfection is no trifle."

Although short of stature, he is tall in character, possessing a subtle humor. His conversation sparkles with the sharp retort. He is religiously honest with his patients. His many kind acts and his love of children are qualities he hides behind a brusque façade. He cherishes his keen analysis of human nature and seldom is he wrong in his appraisals.

A paper by Dr. Burns on an osteoperiosteal chisel indicates one of his technical improvements. A study of over two hundred cases of osteomyelitis published in 1931 shows the importance of that disease at that period and reminds us that therapeutic agents now available have made that infectious disease rare.[2]

Another admirable successor to Dr. Gaenslen, trained close to his elbows, is Dr. Herman W. Wirka. We are happy to salute him as one of our Madison, Wisconsin, products; he was born and raised here and received his B.A. in 1928 and M.D. in 1930 at the University. He became an assistant in orthopedic surgery and has been a successful member of the hospital and Medical School staff ever since, gaining in stature and skill with Drs. Gaenslen and Burns.

I remember him as a Letters and Science student when with his deep resonant voice and his fine sense of the dramatic he assumed many roles with the Wisconsin Players so well that he had difficulty in making the choice between the paths of medicine and the alluring opportunities on the stage. I remember him again as a competent medical student and later as a younger colleague, when he was always ready to put on clinical demonstrations for the classes in medical bacteriology. In those days a patient was not infrequently suffering from acute osteomyelitis. Still later, Dr. Wirka became the ever-dependable orthopedic surgeon who reduced fractures with skill, remedied bad joints, and straightened the backs of his patients, thus winning their everlasting gratitude.

Dr. Wirka is an admirable combination of humility, surgical skill, and deep interest in each patient. To classes or county societies he presents his material with colorful emphasis and dramatic timing, but he does not write papers. Instead he has "written" successfully on the straight backs and useful legs and arms of children, now adults. He has energy and excited interest that carries him through the entire day.

Dr. Wirka is devoted to his family, his church, his patients, and his profession with all too little time left for fishing and other hobbies. Although we are sure he would have done well "on the boards," yet we are happy and grateful that he made what seems to us the correct decision.

RESIDENTS IN ORTHOPEDIC SURGERY THROUGH 1950

1924	Robert E. Burns
1927	Walter Blount
1928	Douglas Gibson
1930	H. Lewis Greene
1932	Malcolm Millar
	Chester C. Shinbach
1933	Raymond M. Baldwin
1934	Herman Wirka
1935	Irving Tuell
1936	John L. Jennings, Jr.
	Robert Montgomery
1937	Peter Midelfart
1938	Charles Ihle
1939	J. Howard Johnson
	E. M. Dessloch
	E. R. Nelson
1940	Vernon C. Turner
1942	William J. Stark
	Henrique A. DeGoes e Vasconcellos
	S. C. Rogers
1943	Luis Lopes
	Jose Machado
1944	Charles Bechtol
	Frederick G. Gaenslen
	Pedro Luis Arias
1945	Wilbur W. Bartels

1946	James W. Brooke
	Richard C. Deming
	James E. Miller
1947	James W. Nellen
	A. E. Culmer
	William I. Norton
1948	Charles W. Christenson
1949	Richard P. Embick
	Norman M. Harris
	Henry I. Okagaki
1950	Jack D. Moore
	Carl A. Stolberg

PLASTIC SURGERY

Dr. George Van Ingen Brown (1862–1948), one of the striking trio of physicians who came from Milwaukee to Madison each week from 1920 on, gradually built up a service in plastic and oral surgery. Immaculate and precise in appearance, in manner, and in his operative techniques, he obtained good results even in operative fields that were far from clean. Asepsis was an engrossing interest with him. He even had his own operating gowns and canvas covers for his shoes. Before the Wisconsin General Hospital was completed, both he and Dr. Gaenslen operated in the Bradley Memorial Hospital.

Dr. Brown was born in St. Paul, Minnesota, in 1862. Initially a dentist, he studied in several institutions, receiving the M.D. degree in 1909 from Marquette University. His professional tasks carried him far afield, and he had patients from practically every state in the country and performed operations also in Canada and in France. He was ingenious in devising operations; the bone flap operation in cleft palate surgery was one of the more successful. Exceedingly meticulous in his work, he was at times explosive if things did not go right. He was a prolific writer and published many articles on harelip and cleft palate. His book on oral diseases and malformations went through several editions.[3] A man of distinction in any group, he received well-merited honors both at home and abroad.[4]

He was a great admirer of Chesapeake Bay dogs and used these dogs hunting in many parts of the country and in Canada, occasionally combining hunting trips with operating duties. He also devoted considerable attention to the Boy Scouts and the educational opportunities this organization gave to our young men.

Dr. Volney Butman Hyslop was Dr. G. V. I. Brown's first resident and his efficient successor in plastic surgery at the Wisconsin Medical School. He took his first two years of medical training here at Wisconsin, completed the work for the M.D. degree at Washington University Medical School (St. Louis) in 1924. He then returned to us and grew up under the meticulous guiding hand of Dr. Brown. Dr. Hyslop developed splendidly in this difficult specialty, and as the senior man approached retirement age, the major load and the mantle fell on the younger shoulders.[5] When Dr. Brown became emeritus professor in 1937–38, Dr. Hyslop was promoted to the full professorship (part-time) in plastic and oral surgery.

To our regret, Dr. Hyslop resigned in 1944 to continue in private practice in Milwaukee. Since Dr. Hyslop left us, plastic surgery has been through the period of this history in the competent hands of Dr. Wayne B. Slaughter.

The University of Wisconsin Medical School has never entered the field of dentistry. When service in that field has been needed, several Madison dentists have provided the necessary aid. In the different decades, the following dentists have served our needs and we are grateful: Samuel Hamilton Chase, Edwin F. Westover, Lester M. Antonius, and Leslie E. Antonius.

RESIDENTS IN PLASTIC SURGERY THROUGH 1950
1924–26 Volney B. Hyslop
1942   Lawrence L. Anderson

GENERAL SURGERY

After Drs. Gaenslen and Brown had instituted surgical teaching and practice in their special areas in the Medical School, there arose the question of the first full-time professor of surgery. All agreed that this appointment was of paramount importance. Much time was spent and many conferences held with prominent surgeons of the country. Admittedly, differences of opinion developed in the faculty. Finally in 1924, Dr. Carl Arthur Hedblom, prominent surgeon at the Mayo Clinic, was chosen. He had had extensive experience. After his early education at Colorado College (B.A., 1907), he received professional training at Harvard Medical School (M.D., 1911) and Massachusetts General Hospital (1911–13). He was professor of surgery at Harvard Medical School in China, 1913–16, and fellow and surgeon at the Mayo Clinic, 1917–24. He was appointed full-time professor of surgery in the University of Wisconsin Medical School in 1924. He was exceptionally powerful physically and had earned a fine reputation as a skilful thoracic surgeon. Unfortunately, he did not fit in well with the opportunities and with some of the faculty members here. After two years,[6] he accepted the position of surgeon-in-chief in the Research and Educational Hospital of the University of Illinois in Chicago. The members of his staff soon left us for other opportunities.

Following Dr. Hedblom's departure, the problem of finding a new professor of surgery was resolved by naming a man whom Dr. Bardeen and the faculty knew well, Dr. Erwin Rudolph Schmidt (1890–1961). He had received his undergraduate training at the University of Wisconsin, completing the B.S. degree and the first two years of medical training in 1913, and had been an assistant in anatomy the following year. He earned the M.D. degree at Washington University Medical School in 1916 in the midst of World War I. He then enjoyed widely varied experience in medicine and surgery — two years in the Army Medical Corps, visits to clinics and studies in several European universities, valuable surgical training under Dr. A. J. Ochsner at Augustana Hospital, Chicago, and two years of private practice in Billings, Montana.

He was appointed professor of surgery in the University of Wisconsin Medical School in 1925 and served in that capacity and as chairman of the department throughout the period of this history and beyond. Dr. Schmidt was completely devoted to his profession; the duties and rewards of his surgical practice were his life. He had no hobbies. He was dedicated to his patients and they in turn almost worshiped him; his bearing on the wards encouraged that attitude. Tall, dignified, assured, benevolent, when he placed his hand on the patient's shoulder, it was a benediction. Of course, his remarks were commonly phrased in words that the patient did not comprehend, so that queries of the patient to the more readily approachable younger associates were frequently embarrassing, for they wondered how much Dr. Schmidt wanted the patient to know.

Dr. Schmidt was a skillful surgeon; his hands, which were truly beautiful, moved with precision. He was a conservative surgeon, frequently preferring to wait and see rather than to use the scalpel immediately. His surgical judgment proved remarkably good. He had a strong aseptic conscience; he wore gloves, even when driving his car. Dr. John Grinde writes in a recent letter:

During my residency in surgery, I once asked Dr. Schmidt if he found his long fingers and slender hands (the typical surgeon's hands in novels) a great advantage. Dr. Schmidt held his novelists' surgical hand out, looked at it and said, "Well, Johnny, I really think the long fingers would be a great thing for urologists because they can't enlarge the incision, but as for surgery, I think much more important is length of thought and depth of knowledge. Watch Joe Gale; his fingers aren't so long, but he sure gets them in the right place fast."

Although Dr. Schmidt was not greatly interested in doing research, he would get up in the middle of the night to perform an operation that he thought necessary. He made rounds every day. His ideal was obviously that of the German *Geheimrat*. The younger men were expected to learn by watching him. The more detailed training of the residents with actual opportunity to operate under direction was an important function that Dr. Gale performed. Dr. Schmidt always stressed to his residents and interns the importance of the basic sciences — anatomy, bacteriology, pathology, physiology. "If you know your basic sciences, you can hardly go wrong in your surgery," was his teaching.

Of his published researches, possibly an early paper on gastric and duodenal ulcers from his European experience was a favorite. He occasionally mentioned an old paper on burns and with Dr. Waters contributed to our knowledge of cyclopropane anesthesia.[7] Like all surgeons, he was interested in the processes of wound healing.

He read widely and enjoyed delving into the history of medicine with several papers for the Miller seminar. He especially appreciated Paracelsus, that fascinating combination of philosopher, early pharmacologist, and mountebank.[8] However, despite the breadth of his interests, Dr. Schmidt was rarely able to communicate such correlations to his students.

He greatly enjoyed his position as head of one of the two great clinical departments and appreciated his professional family. He felt free to make his own decisions and commonly gave similar freedom and support to the younger men.

During World War II, Dr. Schmidt and Dr. Curreri were required to stay here to carry on their surgical and teaching duties while others were permitted to join the armed forces. Gallantry is found not only on the field of battle.

Dr. Kenneth Elroy Lemmer is a true Wisconsin product — Grade A. A native of the state, he took his academic studies here and earned the Wisconsin medical degree in 1930. After an internship at the Medical College of Virginia, he returned for the residency in surgery with Dr. Schmidt. Save for rewarding "brain dusting" expeditions hither and yon and his war service, he has remained here at the University of Wisconsin and attained full professorship in 1954. As the long-time close associate of Dr. Schmidt, he came to resemble him in many ways, especially in his skillful hands, his stress on aseptic technique, and his interest in patient welfare; better organization of his lecture material, including the underlying disturbed physiology, has made him the stronger teacher. He joined with Dr. Gale in the important dog surgery course and, also with Gale, he has devoted time and thought to the direct training of interns and residents. Abdominal surgery has been his major field with ulcerative colitis and primary carcinoma of the liver among his special interests.

He has always been dependable, whether on a difficult surgical case, handling individual human problems, or helping in the organization of the University of Wisconsin Medical Alumni Association. He is a member of the important professional societies and has received well-merited honors both in war and in peace at home and abroad.

Until recently he has been somewhat overshadowed by his chief but he has borne that with good grace. Of his research papers written in the period to 1950, we can cite two, the drainage of the common bile duct with Dr. J. P. Malec and one on carcinoid tumors of the stomach.[9]

The Medical School Alumni Association has had a slow growth, as has the Medical School; Dr. Lemmer has been one of the persistent stalwarts here on the campus in pushing it forward and in stressing donations to the construction of the medical library as the most important project for the alumni. When he can find the time, Dr. Lemmer enjoys and plays a steady game of golf.

Dr. Anthony R. Curreri took his collegiate and his medical courses here at the University of Wisconsin (B.A., 1930; M.A., 1931; M.D., 1933). After an internship at Columbia Hospital in Milwaukee, he returned to the Wisconsin General Hospital for the resident's training in surgery. Save for military leave in the Korean War and professional duties in diverse areas, he has remained at the University as one of the strong members of the department of surgery with advancement to full professorship in 1954.

His enthusiasm, his unfailing good nature, and the nicety of his surgical skill have been strong assets. His pleasant relations with the other hospitals and with the physicians and citizens of the state have been helpful to the Medical School and to the University. He is deeply appreciated by his students, by his peers, by the residents trained in the department, and by his patients.

Of his earlier papers, before he became immersed in the cancer field, most were in the broad area of pulmonary disease and thoracic surgery. One of these has been cited elsewhere; here we shall mention one on successful decortication in chronic empyema and a fine report on mediastinal tumors.[10]

Dr. Curreri has been smilingly aggressive both as a student athlete with boxing gloves and baseball bat as well as later in his professional life. He organizes both his work and his play with skill. In recent years he has kept physically fit with vigorous setting-up exercises and gardening. With his engaging smile and his widely varied associations, he was a most valuable aid to President Fred in obtaining our splendid Memorial Library, that most-needed University building. He helped also in meeting the emotional arguments of the anti-vivisectionists so that animal experimentation could be continued without hampering restrictions. "One man in his time plays many parts."

RESIDENTS IN SURGERY THROUGH 1950

1925	Sidney K. Beigler
1927	Hugh M. Fogo
1929	Karl Friedbacher
	Kurt A. Heinrich
1930	Everett B. Keck
1931	Arthur C. Taylor

1933   Rudolf Howald
       Frank D. Weeks
1934   Kenneth E. Lemmer
1935   Stuart C. Cullen
1936   John L. Keeley
1937   Peter A. Midelfart
       Rudolph J. Noer
1938   John P. Malec
       Carlyle R. Pearson
       Maurice G. Rice
1939   Anthony R. Curreri
       John M. Grinde
       James M. Sullivan
1940   Frederick G. Hidde
       Florence Pettus
1941   Eugene P. Adashek
       Frederick J. Joachim
1942   Reinhold Kanzler
       Dermont W. Melick
       John F. Poser
1943   Otto V. Hibma
1944   James L. Neller
1946   Richard A. Davis
       Cary S. Peabody
       B. Jack Longley
       Forder A. McIver
       Myron A. Myers
       William H. Pollard
1948   Henry A. Szujewski
       John A. Flatley
       Roy B. Larson
1949   George R. Thuerer
       Nicholas G. Maximov
       John T. Mendenhall
       Bertrand W. Meyer
       William P. Young
1950   Edward L. Doermann
       William E. Gilmore
       Lloyd O. Rupe

THORACIC SURGERY

After an extensive residency in surgery under Dr. Ewarts Graham at Barnes Hospital, St. Louis, Dr. Joseph Wasson Gale came here in 1927 to augment our department of surgery. A native of Iowa, he had earned both the B.S. and M.A. degrees at the University of Missouri and the M.D. degree at Washington University in 1924. He became the competent younger member of the surgical team and a leader in thoracic surgery and the study of pulmonary disease. Dr. Gale was the one who early taught the residents in surgery by first permitting them to assist him and then criticizing them, sometimes severely, when they later took over a major position on the team. They were somewhat afraid of his bark, but he did not bite. He and many others have felt that the harsh method is the one that keeps persons on their toes and gets results. Certainly our surgical residents have done well. Dr. Lemmer, a slightly younger member of the surgical staff, recalls those earlier days with appreciation. For many years also, Gale's course in dog surgery, held in the sunny attic of old Science Hall, gave the medical students experience in the elements of surgery, taught them the necessity of delicate handling of fragile tissues, and gave them practice in anesthesia under Dr. Waters.

Dr. Gale contributed significantly to the surgical treatment of pulmonary tuberculosis. With the assistance of Dr. Ralph Waters, an intubation technique of anesthesia was developed, making it possible to anesthetize the normal lung and maintain artificial respiration while permitting surgical procedures on the diseased lung. The number of thoracoplasty operations increased until as many as 250 were performed in a year at the Wisconsin General Hospital. After World War II, more complete pulmonary resections became important in the treatment. Some 7500 patients have had their chest surgery carried on in the Wisconsin General Hospital, mostly by Dr. Gale. The operative mortality has been remarkably low, only 3 per cent. But more important, 90 per cent of the patients treated surgically have been benefited. Dr. Gale's skill soon gave him a position of prominence among thoracic surgeons and earned him well-merited honors. Of his published papers, those on the surgical treatment of pulmonary disease with several associates are noteworthy.[11]

Dr. Gale is a vigorous, aggressive, yet sensitive person; like all good surgeons, he is versatile and prompt in meeting emergencies. His forthright opinions and quick judgments are an integral part of the man who has done so much for so many patients and for the University of Wisconsin Medical School.

He is devoted to outdoor sports, is an ardent huntsman, and enjoys fishing and telling stories about fishing.

UROLOGY

Dr. Ira Roscoe Sisk was for many years our highly successful head of urology; indeed, aside from a few of the early members of the Student Health Service, Dr. Sisk was one of the senior clinical members of our faculty. From Vanderbilt University (M.D., 1916), he joined our staff as an assistant in clinical medicine as early as 1917. After two years in urology at the Mayo Clinic, he began the development of this specialty in Madison and in the Student Health Service.

As soon as the Wisconsin General Hospital was functioning, Dr. Sisk forged ahead and advanced in rank to professor of urology (half-time) by 1930. A benign and cooperative attitude was manifest in his dealings with students, faculty, and patients. He was one of the part-time men who did so much for the Medical School. He built up a considerable bibliography over the years, but our limitations restrict citation to an article on an extensive experimental study in dogs on the transplantation of the ureters to the sigmoid and two on gonococcal infections.[12] Dr. Sisk continued effectively on our staff and in private practice until beyond our historical orbit; he gets much pleasure from his farm in the Verona neighborhood.

Dr. John Brewster Wear (1901–65) came to the University of Wisconsin with a B.A. degree from the University of Texas in 1922 and an M.D. degree from that university's medical school at Galveston in 1926. After an internship at Vanderbilt University Hospital, he became a resident in urology at the Wisconsin General Hospital under Dr. Ira Sisk. His manifest skill brought him rapid advance both in private practice with Dr. Sisk and also in the Wisconsin Medical School, with which he became closely identified throughout his life.[13] He attained full professorship in charge of urology (part-time basis) in 1950.

Dr. Wear worked hard and played hard with success in both of these phases of life. His skill in the difficult field of his choice earned him the outspoken respect of his peers. He was the first to perform a peritoneal dialysis on a human patient in this community. He was also a good teacher; the students liked his staccato one-two-three-four type of teaching. Dr. Wear believed and practiced the old adage that silence is golden; but some elements of medical practice could make him break over this barrier. When surgeons boasted only of their five-year survivals in patients with carcinoma of the prostate gland, he insisted strenuously that they include the dead patients as well and also the period of useful life subsequent to the diagnosis. He urged medical students and residents to know their patients and their personal problems. Any physician who did not show appreciation of the work of nurses, orderlies, and attendants aroused his ire, which could be quite vehement. He was a member of the important professional organizations and enjoyed relaxation in the local social clubs, especially the Maple Bluff Country Club, which provided him with friendly contacts and his favorite sport, golf, and the Madison Club, which gave opportunities for bridge and poker.

RESIDENTS IN UROLOGY THROUGH 1950

1928	John B. Wear
1930	Harold A. O'Brien
1932	Ernest V. Stadel
1933	Earl F. Cummings
1934	C. J. Frick
1937	Palmer Kundert
1938	Otto E. Toenhart
1939	Albert J. Trinkle
1940	Victor Neu
1941	Philip M. Cornwell
	John R. Edwards
	Richard W. Jacobsen
1942	Reinhold Kanzler
	Homer H. Kohler
1944	William W. Leifer
1945	Sidney Hurwitz
1946	Harvey L. Barsch
1947	Frank M. Hilpert
1948	Anton P. Schoenenberger
1950	Norman J. Helland

OPHTHALMOLOGY, RHINOLOGY, OTOLARYNGOLOGY

In 1920, the year of our expansion into several clinical specialties, Dr. Frederick Allison Davis was appointed ophthalmologist in charge of that specialty in the Medical School and was soon advanced to professor of ophthalmology. Dr. Davis was born in 1883 and grew up in Texas. He earned the M.D. degree at the University of Pennsylvania in 1908 and had broad training in ophthalmology and otolaryngology at the New York Eye and Ear Infirmary and also in Philadelphia and Vienna.

In 1925, in response to the urging of Dr. Joseph Evans, Dr. Davis reluctantly accepted the professorship of otolaryngology as well as ophthalmology. The responsibilities of this latter field and of rhinology were gradually shifted to younger men, especially to Dr. Wellwood M. Nesbit, who soon assumed charge of these specialties. Although on a part-time basis, with only the usual nominal salary and commonly with inadequate space, Dr. Davis successfully carried the responsibilities of the clinic, of teaching, and of research.

In order to teach the fundamentals of ophthalmology more effectively, he instituted a short course in the microscopic anatomy and pathology of the eye. The clinical teaching went hand in hand with the didactic instruction, and his work with students, staff, and patients has been greatly appreciated. The highly successful private clinic, of which Dr. Davis has been the head for so many years, has provided both patients and opportunities for the younger men.

Of Dr. Davis' more than twenty published papers, only two can be cited here — a teaching manual on what the general practitioner should know about ophthalmoscopic examination and an extensive and detailed paper on primary tumors of the optic nerve, a phenomenon of Von Recklinghausen's disease.[14]

Dr. Davis' skill as a pianist has delighted both himself and his friends. His home and extensive garden, a short distance from the Old Sauk Road, have always been a haven for his family and his friends.

Dr. Eugene Ezra Neff (1890–1949) joined Dr. Davis and the Medical School in 1924. He was born in Virginia, received the B.A. degree from Emory and Henry College and his M.D. degree from the University of Virginia Medical School in 1916, an institution to which he remained highly devoted. Immediate service in the Medical Corps of the United

States Army for two years and graduate studies in the New York Eye and Ear Infirmary from 1919–22 gave him an excellent professional basis for his appointments with Dr. Davis and the University of Wisconsin Medical School. He served with high success as a member of the Davis-Neff Clinic and the Medical School until his untimely death in 1949.

Dr. Neff was a rare blithe spirit, a gay optimistic physician whose cordial greetings resounded through the halls and gave courage to the downhearted. He gave to all a splendid example of the art of medicine well supported by extensive knowledge, experience, and warm personal interest. He was not interested in research beyond the constant need to study the problems of each patient. He was especially aware of the opportunities to practice preventive medicine in his specialty.

Dr. Peter Alexander Duehr received his academic and first two years of medical training at the University of Wisconsin (B.A., 1926; M.A., 1927) and his M.D. degree at Rush Medical College of the University of Chicago in 1929. After an internship here, he continued in ophthalmology, advancing consistently to full professorship (part-time) in 1953. With Dr. Duehr, as with many of our so-called part-time appointees, his devotion to his patients both in and out of the hospital and to the students has always been paramount. His operative skills have brought him an excellent reputation throughout the state. He has become especially proficient in operations for cataract and for detached retina. One of his early published papers summarizes the factors and the results in 104 consecutive cases of retinal detachment.[15]

His quiet calm competence and his manifest kindliness have given confidence to his patients at critical times and have endeared him to colleagues and students. His mode of life has not given him much opportunity for interests beyond his profession, but he did at an earlier period have a superb rose garden.

Dr. Wellwood M. Nesbit (1891–1953) earned his M.D. degree at Rush Medical College in 1917, took his intern year at Presbyterian Hospital, Chicago, and specialized in otolaryngology at Washington University Medical School. He then came to Madison to enter private practice in his specialty. In 1925 he was appointed by the staff of the Medical School to serve in his fields with Dr. Frederick A. Davis.

Increasingly, the responsibility for ear, nose, and throat fell on the shoulders of the younger man, and the catalogue of 1930–31 states that

Dr. Nesbit was in charge of rhinology, laryngology, and otology. Assured, competent, handsome, and a good mixer, Dr. Nesbit promptly won an important place for himself in otolaryngology in the Medical School and in the city. Early he made use of the bronchoscope for removing foreign bodies from the bronchus. He was the competent clinician rather than an investigator. Of his researches we shall cite one study made with Drs. Middleton and Paul on congenital aplasia of the lung.[16]

From his early boyhood days, the lure of the land continued to grip Dr. Nesbit, and he enjoyed the ownership of a farm outside Madison. Another facet of his many-sided personality is shown by his friendship with several contemporary painters and the work of the prominent men of its midwestern school.

Dr. Mark E. Nesbit also shared in the duties of the eye, ear, nose, and throat clinics and in the teaching from the early thirties until after our period. He and his older brother worked well as a team and shared many of the same affable attributes. Later, Mark began to specialize in ophthalmology and resigned from the University to restrict himself to private practice in that field in Madison.

RESIDENTS IN OPHTHALMOLOGY, RHINOLOGY, AND
OTOLARYNGOLOGY THROUGH 1950

1926	M. J. Bach
1931	William A. Werrell
	Harry McGrath
1932	Benjamin Brindley
1933	Merrill O. Eiel
1934	Peter A. Duehr
1935	James Dollard
1936	Hugh Autrey
1937	Ralph W. Stevens
1938	Ray L. Allison
1939	Morton Cutler
1940	Claude Miller
1941	Edward G. Schott
1942	Jack D. Brownfield
	Charles M. Polan
	Milton G. Radewan
1944	John M. Wilson
1945	Clifford D. Hogenson

1946	George K. Kambara
1947	Robert M. Hansen
1948	George B. Corcoran, Jr.
	William C. Randolph
	Charles R. Taborsky
	Levon D. Yazujian
1949	Robert C. Randolph
	Robert E. Hawkins
1950	Richard H. Brodhead

NEUROSURGERY

Dr. Theodore Charles Erickson was appointed associate professor of surgery at the University of Wisconsin Medical School in 1941 to take on the heavy responsibilities of his special field, neurosurgery. Dr. Erickson had received his academic and early medical training at the University of Minnesota (B.S., 1928; M.A., 1929; M.D., 1931) and continued his medical studies at the University of Pennsylvania Hospital, 1931–33. He then had extensive experience in neurosurgery with Dr. Wilder Penfield at McGill University, 1934–41, earning the Ph.D. degree in 1939 with a scholarly experimental thesis on the nature and spread of epileptic discharge. His broad background, his critical approach to the complex problems in his field, and his skillful hands brought him prompt acceptance by colleagues, patients, and students.

Dr. Erickson's period at Wisconsin extends well beyond our purview, so we must restrict our references to his important work with Penfield and that at Wisconsin on epileptiform-like seizures, contributions that are typical of one of his major interests.[17]

RESIDENTS IN NEUROLOGICAL SURGERY THROUGH 1950

1943	Joseph F. Charest
1946	Henry M. Suckle
1949	Richard H. Retter

CHEMOSURGERY

Dr. Frederic E. Mohs was one of the three original Bowman fellows when, in 1935, plans for using the Bowman Fund for cancer research were initiated. Dr. Mohs, a native of Wisconsin, took both his undergraduate and medical studies here at the University and received the M. D. degree in 1934. While still a second-year medical student he began studies on malignant tumors of the rat as a research assistant of Dr. M. F. Guyer, chairman of the department of zoology. Upon Mohs' return to Wisconsin, after an internship at Portland, Oregon, he continued a life devoted to cancer studies. As a result of his early investigations, he published in 1941 two important papers, one with Dr. Guyer on a pre-excisional fixation of malignant tissues with several escharotic chemicals, of which zinc chloride proved the most effective agent. A related investigation in this field that he made his own is on chemosurgery, a microscopically controlled method of cancer excision.[18]

Dr. Mohs states in his monograph in this field that many persons, beginning possibly with Sir Humphrey Davy, have used zinc chloride and other reagents for their caustic action on tissues. His own important and highly successful contribution is the painstaking microscopic control of the excision, with continuation of the treatment and the microscopic studies until the "silent" extensions that are not detectable clinically have been removed. The number of five-year cures, as recorded in 1948, is remarkable — 96.2 per cent of 291 cases of basal cell carcinoma and 84.4 per cent of 136 cases of squamous cell carcinoma. Obviously the method is applicable only to accessible growths. It may be used also in the treatment of benign tumors and in a variety of skin infections.[19]

Dr. Mohs' meticulous microscopic attention to the details of the technique, and his quiet appreciation of the human factors involved have earned him the important position as head and associate professor of chemosurgery in the Medical School and the devoted appreciation of his many patients. His outpatient clinic is thronged. In recent years he has been training a number of younger physicians to specialize in chemosurgery.

Dr. Mohs goes quietly but efficiently about his professional duties without commotion. "Golf takes too much daylight time," he says; but he likes to putter in his garden and in his shop with power saw and lathe and he takes time occasionally for a spin on the lake in his motor boat.

22   Department of Obstetrics and Gynecology

If a pregnant woman be attacked by erysipelas of the womb, it is fatal.

Hippocrates

With the development of the four-year Medical School, the needs in obstetrics and gynecology became immediate. To meet these, Drs. Carl S. Harper and Edwin F. Schneiders were appointed first as associates and later as assistant professors in these fields. Both of these men have continued on the staff until well beyond the period of this history. However, in the case of Dr. Schneiders, there was an interim after 1928 when he did not serve with the Medical School because he thought that abuses existed in assigning certain patients to the "clinic" category.

Dr. Carl Harper, a native of Wisconsin and a strong athlete, especially in basketball, took his bachelor's degree and the first two years of medical training here at the University and completed his work for the medical degree in 1916 at the University of Pennsylvania. He has had wide experience in hospitals in Brooklyn, New York, and Philadelphia, as well as those of Madison, and an extensive practice in Madison. He has brought many Wisconsin babies into the world, and his gynecological services have helped many patients. He has made studies in heredity and in sterility,[1] but states that he enjoyed most his contacts with the students. They in turn appreciated the direct vigor of the man and his teaching.

Dr. Schneiders is also a native of Wisconsin and did his undergraduate work and his first two years of medicine here. Like Dr. Harper, he was an athlete, a pitcher on the baseball team. His last two years in medicine were at Harvard, where he earned his M.D. degree in 1921.

179

He was associated with the gas warfare service here during World War I and in that period took a master's degree in pathology with Dr. Bunting. He has signed an incredible number of birth certificates, but his greater interest has been in gynecological surgery.[2] In St. Mary's Hospital and throughout the city, Dr. Schneiders has been a potent force for good medical practice and helpful collaboration. We were happy when he came back to work with us at a period beyond this history.

Dr. John Warton Harris (1891–1955) became professor of obstetrics and gynecology in the University of Wisconsin and head of the services and teaching in those fields in 1928. A warmhearted southerner born in Reedsville, North Carolina, January 12, 1891, he attended the University of North Carolina, obtaining a bachelor of arts degree in 1911 and the master's degree in 1912. He then went to Johns Hopkins University, receiving the M.D. degree in 1916. He became the devoted disciple of the eminent obstetrician, Dr. J. Whitridge Williams. Except for one year at Yale, Dr. Harris remained at Johns Hopkins for twelve years progressing through the various levels of increasing responsibility until 1928 when Dr. Bardeen persuaded him to come here. He promptly became the active, colorful chairman of the newly established department of obstetrics and gynecology.

Dr. Harris had a flare for spicy phrases that stuck in the mind of the student — allegedly, even when the student was asleep. He was knowledgeable, exacting, and perceptive; he taught well at all levels. He had high ideals and standards of probity; he was generous and kind, indeed a lovable person. It was a pleasure to sit with him at lunch. He created an atmosphere devoid of haste and rush; these demons went out the window when John took his seat at the head of the table in the cafeteria.

The students enjoyed Dr. Harris' colorful remarks. Here are some gathered together by Dr. Curtis Lund, one of his excellent residents.[3] His list of superlatives frequently included "quintessence of asininity or stupidity," "100% zero (or nothing)," and "abysmal jackass." He also used picturesque bits of speech, such as "shadbellied" and "predestined Presbyterianism." His comparisons included such comments as "so fat she looked like a broken barrel of molasses on a stool," "as likely as hot ice cream," "as likely as a heat stroke in January in Madison," "as futile as an attempt to empty Lake Mendota with a teaspoon," "as futile as my attempts to perform a ballet." He consoled young mothers, heavy with child, by reminding them that however cumbersome they might become, he was permanently larger and heavier, and he enjoyed making fun of his large dimensions.

The bacteriology of infections in parturient women was Dr. Harris' chief field of research, and these studies were carried out at Johns Hopkins before he came to Wisconsin. He described a type of puerperal sepsis fairly common then in Baltimore caused by viridans (alpha hemolytic) streptococci or by non-hemolytic organisms, not a fulminating type of the disease as caused by the beta hemolytic streptococci. These cases are significant in the total picture of puerperal sepsis.[4] Dr. Harris did little research at Wisconsin. One paper with Dr. Waters on carbon dioxide and oxygen in obstetric anesthesia may be cited.[5]

Aside from his professional activities, Dr. Harris' interests were his home and family, his church, and his garden. He stimulated his associates; residents in the department have carried on excellently both at the University of Wisconsin and in other institutions.

One of Dr. Harris' active associates, Dr. Ralph Campbell, came to the University after college studies at Dartmouth (B.S., 1920), a medical degree from Northwestern (1922), and further work in obstetrics and gynecology at Johns Hopkins and McGill Medical School. Always good-natured and smiling, prompt with a joke, he establishes easy relations not only with his patients, but also with their families. He is both genial and jovial. Dr. Campbell continued to grow in the field of his specialties, attaining the rank of full professor in 1946. Of his published papers, several on menstrual irregularities and sterility have advanced our knowledge in these clinical mysteries. One of his favorite studies was done with Dr. Pohle and showed favorable results over a period of years in the use of deep X-ray in experimental tuberculosis in dogs.[6] As with so many of the faculty, golf is his major outdoor sport.

Dr. Madeline J. Thornton, the second resident in obstetrics here at Wisconsin, 1929–31, was, according to her chief, Dr. Harris, "the best one I ever had." Her education followed excellent paths: Syracuse University (B.A., 1923), Johns Hopkins Medical School (M.D., 1927), and an internship in medicine at the Research and Educational Hospital, Chicago, 1929. Dr. Thornton treasures her words, is shy, reluctant to speak, but prompt in her professional decisions when speed is desirable, and she is skillful in accomplishing her objectives. A favorite among her published papers is a controlled study of the use of vaginal tampons for the absorption of menstrual discharge.[7]

Dr. Thornton has earned the confidence of students, staff, and her many patients; she has achieved consistent advance in responsibilities and academic rank. Her hobbies are music and her stamp collection.

RESIDENTS IN OBSTETRICS AND GYNECOLOGY
THROUGH 1950

1930	Everett Keck
1931	Madeline J. Thornton
1933	Herbert M. Aitken
1934	Wilford Risteen
1936	Ronald Martin
1937	Russell Muntz
	John Parks
1938	Gordon Peterson
1939	Curtis Lund
1940	Robert Woodhull
1941	Gerald Brown
1942	John H. Rendok
1943	Nan Denholm
	John Morton
1944	William R. Knight
1945	Alice D. Watts
1946	John Boersma
	Horacio Eyzaguirre-Huici
1947	Jerome Maas
1948	Robert Barter
	Cary Peabody
1949	Howard J. Tatum
1950	William Luetke

23 Department of Radiology

We all labour against our own cure, for death is the cure of all diseases.

Thomas Browne, RELIGIO MEDICI

In thinking of the early days of studies with roentgen rays in the Medical School, older members of the faculty will remember with pleasure the brothers Hodges, both Paul C. and Fred J., and their work with Dr. Eyster and Dr. Bardeen on heart size and cardiophysiology. Paul had a varied early career with several degrees at irregular intervals because of jobs well done; he earned his M.D. degree at Washington University Medical School (St. Louis) in 1918 and a Ph.D. in physiology at Wisconsin in 1924. After several years working in roentgenology at Peking Union Medical School, he returned to this country in 1927 to carry on with distinction his clinical studies and teaching in this field at the University of Chicago.

Dr. Fred Jenner Hodges took his undergraduate studies and first two years of medical training at Wisconsin, completed the work for the medical degree at Washington University (St. Louis) in 1919, and continued there for a residency in pathology. He returned to Wisconsin in 1921 with an appointment in the department of physiology. Subsequently, he developed the courses in radiology in our Medical School and the clinical work with X-rays both at the Wisconsin General Hospital and at St. Mary's Hospital. Only one of his early papers can be cited; a study with Dr. Eyster on transverse cardiac diameter in man.[1] In 1931, Dr. Hodges, to our regret, went to the University of Michigan to accept the chair in radiology there.

In 1928, Dr. Ernst Albert Pohle (1885–1965), a medical graduate from Frankfurt, Germany, became the first professor of radiology at the

183

University of Wisconsin. Dr. Pohle came to us from the University of Michigan, where he had been in the department of radiology for some years and had also earned a Ph.D. in biophysics. He was an active and prolific contributor to his field, both in basic and in clinical research, with approximately a hundred titles in his complete bibliography. His studies of the effect of radiation on normal tissues, especially the heart, and on the healing of wounds, were highly regarded.[2] He installed the first radon plant in this area for the preparation of radon seeds which were widely used at that time in the treatment of a variety of malignant conditions. In addition to his numerous papers, he was the editor of three well-regarded and voluminous textbooks;[3] he especially valued the one on clinical roentgen therapy, the field of his major interest. Dr. Pohle was precise in his own studies, in his therapeutic practice, and in his teaching. He trained many residents, about twenty-five up to 1950, who have continued to maintain the high standards of their teacher.

Dr. Pohle did not give much of his time to hobbies, but he did enjoy roaming the fields of Wisconsin and during his more active years was an ardent huntsman.

Dr. Lester Warner Paul received his academic and early medical training at the University of Minnesota (B.S., 1922; M.D., 1925). After his internship, he enjoyed several years of private practice before coming to the Wisconsin General Hospital in the department of radiology in 1930. Happily, he has remained here building up with Dr. Pohle a splendidly complete service in clinical radiology well grounded on fundamental studies. While Dr. Pohle generally handled the therapeutic problems, Dr. Paul's forte has been his diagnostic acumen and knowledge, astounding his fellow physicians with the accuracy of his diagnoses from the X-ray films. Of his many publications, we may cite in our restricted story one paper on the roentgen diagnosis of carcinoma of the pancreas, one with Dr. Pohle on solitary myeloma of bone, and two papers on pulmonary adenomatosis, the first with Dr. Gorton Ritchie and the second with Dr. J. H. Juhl.[4]

Dr. John Harold Juhl came here as resident in radiology in 1946; his major accomplishments in the field have therefore occurred after the period of this chronicle. He received both his academic and early medical training at the University of Michigan (B.A., 1936; M.D., 1940). He immediately became involved in war work and then served in the Navy until he came to Madison, where he has built up a fine reputation in the diagnostic field of radiology. His faculty associates have found him especially cooperative and a good administrator; the students appreciate his well-organized instruction.

RESIDENTS IN RADIOLOGY THROUGH 1950

1932	Frank G. Drischel
1934	A. Russell Anderson
	Emil M. Shebesta
1937	Helene Boyer
	C. M. Lightner
1938	Samuel R. Beatty
1940	John McAneny
1941	Leonard Long
	Maurice G. Richter
1942	B. Kenneth Lovell
	Clarence S. Youngstrom
1944	Roland R. Benson
	Evelyn Siris
1945	Elizabeth Clark
1946	James A. Morton
1947	Carol Tomlinson
1948	William W. Moir
	Irving Weissman
1949	Ralph C. Frank
	John H. Juhl
	Robert C. Schmitz
1950	Marvin N. Golper

24 Department of Anesthesiology

OTHELLO

Dr. Ralph Milton Waters enjoyed this quotation; in fact, he enjoyed keenly the early history of anesthesia. Indeed, he enjoyed all history and life itself. He played such an important part in our Medical School and in the development of his field that one fumes at the necessary spatial limitations.

During the presidency of Glenn Frank, introduction of prominent new faculty became a part of the first general faculty meeting of the year. Dean Bardeen in his characteristic amiable mumble introduced Dr. Waters, saying that the faculty was not commonly selected for skill in putting people to sleep, but in the case of Dr. Waters that was to be his major function.

From a family farm in Ohio, to a small academy, to Adelbert College of Western Reserve University (B.A., 1907), to the school of medicine of that university (M.D., 1912), to the German Hospital in Cleveland, Ralph Waters climbed well, earning not only his education but much of his maintenance and considerable independence of mind. He began the general practice of medicine in Sioux City, Iowa, in the spring of 1913. Some of Waters' own writing gives us the following account of the practice of medicine in that area and period and his own change from general practice to the field of anesthesia in which he performed so splendidly.

When I came to Wisconsin in 1927, my own background for a career in anesthesia was scanty indeed. Perhaps I was fortunate in that, in the United States, the medical profession had paid little attention to anesthesia, in contrast to Great Britain where administration of anesthetics had been considered a function of the medical profession since the days of John Snow in the mid-1800's. An added factor was possibly the fact that my school days had been thickly overlaid with the necessity of earning most of my keep along the way. This meant that, as a medical student in Cleveland, I had served as night orderly, student helper and extern in various laboratories and hospitals. Since individuals such as these served (in most operating rooms throughout the country at the beginning of the 20th century, even in the great medical centers) as the administrator of most of the anesthetics, it was my opportunity to begin an interest in anesthetics early in my career. My first venture in the practice of medicine was in a Missouri Valley town where there were about a hundred physicians, some ninety-five of whom were professed surgeons. None were anesthetists. The chap with the fewest patients of his own was the most likely to be chosen as the anesthetist for the day. After three years of part-time interest in anesthesia in Sioux City therefore, I gained courage to have cards printed with Practice limited to Anesthesia following my name. That was in 1916. The opportunity of a move to Kansas City came in 1923. The great majority of anesthetics in Kansas City in 1923 were administered by physicians who specialized, more or less, in such work. It was a happy change for me over anything I had experienced before that time. It was obvious that, if the technics of surgery and anesthesia were to improve in the future, medical students must be allowed to learn some of the fundamentals of physiology and pharmacology related to anesthesia along with the technical facility necessary to apply such fundamental knowledge.[1]

Dr. Waters delights in telling of his visit to Madison and the Medical School in 1926, his chats with Drs. Evans, Bardeen, and Schmidt about the establishment of anesthesia on a more scientific basis, and the cordial meetings in the pharmacology laboratories with Arthur Loevenhart and Chauncey Leake. Their investigations with some of the drugs used in anesthesia were known to him, and it was the possibility of further laboratory studies that induced Dr. Waters to accept the position here in charge of anesthesia in the department of surgery.[2] He has told me that he came here especially to work with Dr. Leake and was chagrined when in a year or two Leake accepted a position at the University of California. Dr. Waters describes one of their first experiments in the use of CO_2 and varying concentrations of oxygen. After Dr. Loevenhart had asserted, "You have gone too far. That dog is dead and will never breathe again," Dr. Waters brought the dog back to normal respiration by ventilation with pure oxygen. "The CO_2 came down to normal, the pulse and blood pressure came back to near normal, and Leake and I went on with our experiment."[3]

As Dr. Waters stated in an article in 1948, his objectives at Wisconsin remained as they had been in the beginning: "(1) to provide the best possible service to patients of the institution; (2) to teach what is known of the principles of anesthesiology to all candidates for the medical degree; (3) to help long-term graduate students not only to gain a fundamental knowledge of the subject and to master the art of administration, but also to learn as much as possible of effective methods of teaching; and (4) to accompany these efforts with the encouragement of as much cooperative investigation as is consistent with achieving the first three objectives." [4]

In the more than a hundred published papers in Dr. Waters' bibliography, we find studies on many of the important anesthetic drugs, including hypnotics and sedatives. This breadth of interest is characteristic of the man, as is also the intensive study of the drugs of his choice.

It is not possible in this brief survey to do justice to the researches of Dr. Waters and his associates. Only a few areas and still fewer papers can be cited. Back in his Iowa days in Sioux City (1924), Waters developed the soda lime filter for absorption of carbon dioxide during the time the expired gases are passing through it. This differed little from the "to and fro absorber" of today that has proved so economical in the use of anesthetic agents.[5] When cyclopropane was suggested for use as an anesthetic in 1928, it was carefully studied in the pharmacological laboratory at Wisconsin before it was used on the first patient in 1930. Waters' summary of the results with cyclopropane, presented before the British Medical Association in 1936, is considered a masterpiece.[6] His work with Dr. Tatum on barbiturates and studies with Leake on the anesthetic properties of carbon dioxide rank high on his impressive bibliography.[7] The thorough study of endotracheal anesthesia, including also the splendid monographs on that subject by Dr. Noel A. Gillespie, have taught many the advantages of this method and the types of cases in which it is most useful.[8] Ever and always, Dr. Waters stressed meticulous records of the complete anesthetic history that eventually grew into a punched-card system kept up assiduously by Dr. Gillespie.

Collaborative researches among physiology and pharmacology and the clinical departments were begun by Dr. Waters. The atmosphere has always been informal, friendly yet critical.

Years of investigation on the old controversial anesthetic, chloroform, were initiated by Waters and later published in a monograph under his editorship. In the acknowledgements is this statement: "Those who were mainly responsible for writing this report are E. B. Cohen, N. A. Gillespie, L. E. Morris, O. S. Orth, F. J. Pohle, and J. L. Sims." In the preface of the book, we find this modest disclaimer: "Personally, I feel much like the fly sitting on the axle of the chariot wheel and exclaiming 'what a dust do I raise,' since my own contribution to this effort has been minimal in the extreme. I am most grateful to everyone mentioned in the book and to many others for accomplishing work which I myself had long hoped but neglected to do." [9]

Dr. Waters' teaching of the regular medical students as well as residents and those intending to specialize has been on a high plane of appreciative criticism. The many professional guests in the department from foreign lands as well as from the United States have been guests in his welcoming home.

Dr. Waters had few hobbies. His professional duties, his house and garden, and his wide reading, especially in history and biography, absorbed him. He was deeply interested in the development and in the personal welfare of his younger associates. A warm close relationship existed in the growing anesthesiology family, which became international in its extent. A good example of Ralph Waters' terse, humorous comments comes from the biography of Waters by his associate, Noel Gillespie: "I sat with him once at a meeting. At the end of one paper, he withdrew his pipe from his mouth for the time necessary to remark, 'However thin he slices it, it is still baloney.' " [10] Dr. Waters, full of good works, rich in merited honors, loved and admired as friend and teacher by students and colleagues, retired with all sail set at a youthful sixty-six.

Dr. Noel Alexander Gillespie (1904–55) came to the University of Wisconsin in 1938 from Oxford University and London Hospital Medical College after several years as anesthetist at London Hospital. A high degree of mutual appreciation developed between his chief, Dr. Waters, and Dr. Gillespie. Gillespie's biographical story of Dr. Waters has charm of style and personal detail. I have used it liberally as a source; unfortunately it is too long to take the place of the chapter in this more general history.

Dr. Gillespie's major contributions here were his persistent efforts to maintain superior, detailed records on each patient with annual reports for the department and his splendid monograph on endotracheal anesthesia. This scholarly work went through two editions (1941 and 1948) and a translation into German; it continues to receive appropriate citations.

Dr. Gillespie embodied the characteristic broad interests of the honor students from Oxford and the more leisurely approach to the problems of daily living that our British neighbors still retain to a considerable degree. Gillespie was interested in music, a lover of Bach; he had a splendid collection of records, enjoyed the out-of-doors. He was deeply religious and had rather rare spiritual qualities. He spent two years with Albert Schweitzer in his missionary hospital in Africa. His fine appreciations and interests were assets to the department and the University. His early death in his fifties was a loss to friends and to society.[11]

Dr. Oswald Sidney Orth (1906–64) had a varied and productive career in physiology, pharmacology, and anesthesiology with some seventy published studies. After graduating from the University of Illinois with the B.S. degree in 1929 and spending several years as a graduate assistant in physiology there, he came to Wisconsin as instructor in physiology in 1936. Vigorous and fertile in ideas, Dr. Orth earned the Ph.D. degree in physiology in 1939 and the M.D. degree in 1942. In 1942, he left the department of physiology for that of pharmacology and by 1948 attained full professorship and chairmanship of that department. In 1948, also, he received a joint appointment as professor in the department of anesthesiology, the field of many of his investigations. The next year, when Dr. Waters retired, after a brief interlude during which Dr. Alexander M. MacKay served as acting chairman of the department, Dr. Orth became the active head of anesthesiology and continued to encourage the collaboration of members of the department with men in the underlying sciences and with the clinicians. This collaboration resulted in scholarly papers in physiology and in anesthesiology on new and old hydrocarbons with their action on the heart, on the liver, and on the kidneys. Cyclopropane as one of the new anesthetic agents and chloroform as one of the old were studied intensively. The detailed investigations on the use of chloroform were gathered together in a monograph under the editorship of Dr. Waters. The studies with trichlorethylene must also be cited.[12]

In addition to or as an integral part of his professional duties Dr. Orth shed the light of his happy disposition on all those around him.

His ready smile and his interest in the immediate personal problems of the student, the patient, or friend became a vital part of the life of the department and the Medical School. He and his wife were devoted to roses; their extensive, beautiful rose garden was a labor of love and many hours. It earned merited prizes and was a delight to their many friends. The sudden death of Dr. Orth in 1954 while still young and active came as a shocking blow to his widely scattered friends and associates.[13]

RESIDENTS IN ANESTHESIOLOGY THROUGH 1950

1928	Amy Littig Damm
1929	John Moffitt
1930	Albert J. Wineland
1932	Martha Kohl
	David Treweek
1933	William B. Neff
	Emery A. Rovenstine
1934	John A. Stiles
1935	Malcolm O. Burns
	Ivan B. Taylor
1936	Perry Volpitto
1937	F. A. Alexander
	Virginia Apgar
1938	James H. Bennett
	Hubert Hathaway
1939	William H. Cassels
	M. Digby Leigh
	Barindra N. Sircar
1940	Harvey C. Slocum
	Torsten Gordh
1941	W. Allen Conroy
	Robert D. Dripps
	James M. Foerster
	Noel A. Gillespie
	Ferdinand C. Jacobson
	Clayton Wangeman
1942	Howard Ausherman
	Norma B. Bowles

	Richard Foregger
	Malcolm H. Hawk
	Austin Lamont
1943	Jane M. Moir
	Adolph Shor
1944	Merel H. Harmel
	Bryce K. Ozanne
1945	Milton Davis
	Rosaline L. Wilhelm
1946	Simpson S. Burke, Jr.
	Franklin M. Dowiasch
	Luis H. Bouroncle
	Olle F. Friberg
	Jose Guerra
	Alfredo Pernin
1947	William F. Cormak
	Donald R. Kindschi
	Sven E. Nilsson
	Ronald A. Simpson
	Robert M. Wylde
1948	Willard D. Bennett
	Lucien E. Morris
	Darwin D. Waters
	Carlos P. Parsloe
1949	Dorothy Wittman Betlach
	Karl G. Dhüner
	Jone J. Wu
1950	Ann Bardeen
	Max Baumeister, Jr.
	Gordon M. Garnett
	Jocelyn I. Robb
	Larry H. Hogan
	Betty J. Bamforth

25 Wisconsin General Hospital

A Memorial to Those Who Served the Country in the World War

Erected in Gratitude by the People of the State of Wisconsin.

Bronze plaques with these memorial inscriptions were appropriately placed on either side of the main entrance of the Wisconsin General Hospital, which was officially opened with ceremony on April 29, 1924. This dignified Italian Renaissance structure, with its lovely sunny second-floor loggia and its porches at both east and west ends, was designed by the state architect Arthur Peabody and his staff. For years, Dean Bardeen had been studying hospitals and medical school plants throughout the country.[1] He had broad ideas and Dr. Evans had special appreciation of the finer needs of the physician-nurse-patient relationship. It was with their constant advice that Mr. Peabody and his associate, Frank Moulton, worked so successfully.

The history of the difficulties and final success in obtaining funds for the construction of the hospital has been told in an earlier chapter. The hearty support of this memorial project by the Wisconsin Department of the American Legion should be appreciated. The total amount appropriated for a hospital building, for a residence for nurses, and for equipment was $1,350,000. Additional sums were appropriated for the purchase of land.

The Regents decided on the location of the hospital on University Avenue between Randall Avenue and Charter Street only after much deliberation and consultation. As expressed by Dean Bardeen, "This site lies midway between the collegiate campus and the grounds of the College of Agriculture. . . . We are thus assured of the most advantageous physical relationships between other university departments and the medical school and hospitals." Dr. Bardeen consistently stressed this

193

geographic proximity as providing a distinct advantage over institutions where the medical school and hospital are remote from the main university. He and all members of the early faculty greatly valued the ease of cooperation and consultation thus provided.

The University catalogue has commonly presented a summary statement of the establishment of the hospital, an outline of the major purposes, and its services to patients. Below is a copy from the catalogue of 1934–35, ten years after the hospital was opened.

STATE OF WISCONSIN GENERAL HOSPITAL
R. C. Buerki, Superintendent

The State of Wisconsin General Hospital is established in connection with the Medical School of the University of Wisconsin. The University Infirmary and the Mary Cornelia Bradley Memorial Hospital, previously established, are integral parts of the Hospital (Sec. 36.21, Stat. 1923). The new Children's Orthopedic Hospital (Sec. 36.32, Stat. 1929) is closely affiliated.

The main hospital building is designed as a memorial to those who served in the World War. It was built and equipped from the balance in the Service Recognition Fund (Chapter 20, Spl. S., 1920).

The chief purposes of the hospital are defined as follows: (1) Primarily for the care of persons afflicted with a malady, deformity, or ailment of a nature which probably can be remedied by hospital service and treatment, who would be unable otherwise to secure such care. (2) For such instruction of medical students, physicians, and nurses and for such scientific research as will promote the welfare of the patients committed to its care and assist in the application of science to the alleviation of human suffering (Sec. 36.31, Stat. 1923).

In addition, a limited number of patients able to pay for care are also admitted upon reference. The hospital is primarily interested in the type of patient who is unable to pay for hospital care and who can be benefited by care. All types of cases are accepted at the hospital with the exception of frank pulmonary tuberculosis. These cases, it is felt, can best be treated in the local sanatoria and as soon as a patient who has been admitted to the hospital is diagnosed as such he is recommended for transfer. During the last ten years over 50,000 different patients coming from all sections of the state have received treatment at the State of Wisconsin General Hospital. The present bed capacity of the hospitals is over 600.

The new Orthopedic Hospital has increased the number of orthopedic patients that can be hospitalized at the University. In this unit adequate facilities are provided not only for the actual medical and surgical care necessary, but also classroom space for general education and occupational therapy. The hospital cooperates with the local schools for crippled children throughout the state by returning the patient to his community as early as possible, thereby reducing the cost of care to both state and county.

This synopsis of the detailed statutes does not make clear that the "public patients" must satisfy the county judge that the costs to be assigned — one-half to the county and one-half to the state — are a legitimate public charge. The special rate "clinic patients," on the other hand, are admitted upon recommendation of the family physician. This physician should, therefore, be satisfied that the patient can pay the established hospital rate, but that additional professional fees would work a serious hardship. Since the interpretation of these provisions depends on human judgment, differences of opinion have occurred. At times, a few practicing physicians have felt that the state-supported institution has unjustly interfered with private practice, resulting in grievances brought before the county or the state medical societies. In order to broaden the type of patients for teaching purposes and to provide additional revenue for the hospital, the need for permitting some private practice among the faculty has commonly been recognized.

The privilege of private patient consultation has therefore been granted by the hospital administrative committee upon the recommendation of the chairman of the department concerned. It is granted only to established staff members and on the basis of merit alone. . . . Private patients are able to pay full costs of care both hospital and professional. They are admitted on reference from their family physician. . . .

In addition to these classes of patients, honorably discharged veterans of any United States war may be admitted at a special statutory rate including professional services. Emergency patients are those admitted to meet some special immediate need.

All students in the University who pay an infirmary fee are entitled to care at the Student Infirmary under the charge of the members of the Student Health Service. By statute, the infirmary is made a part of the Wisconsin General Hospital.

The "Outpatient Clinic" is designed for the diagnosis and treatment of conditions which do not require bed care. . . . Outpatients are classified as public, special rate (clinic), and private, and they pay the registration and service charges required of each classification.[2]

The major portion of the fundamental teaching of the clinical branches of medicine is conducted in the Wisconsin General Hospital and the related hospitals of the medical center. The Wisconsin and the Madison Boards of Health cooperate willingly in the practical instruction of the medical students. Collaboration with other hospitals of the city has always been important and is now becoming increasingly fruitful.

All the services of the hospital must be self-supporting, and the Regents are required to make a detailed report of income and expenditures. Summary figures prepared for the thirtieth anniversary of the opening of the hospital (1924–54) showed that it had provided a total of 4,809,158 hospital patient days, of which 3,463,178 were for public patients. The total revenue of the hospital had been $37,853,288.94, and the total

PER DIEM INCOME AND EXPENSE
1924-1954

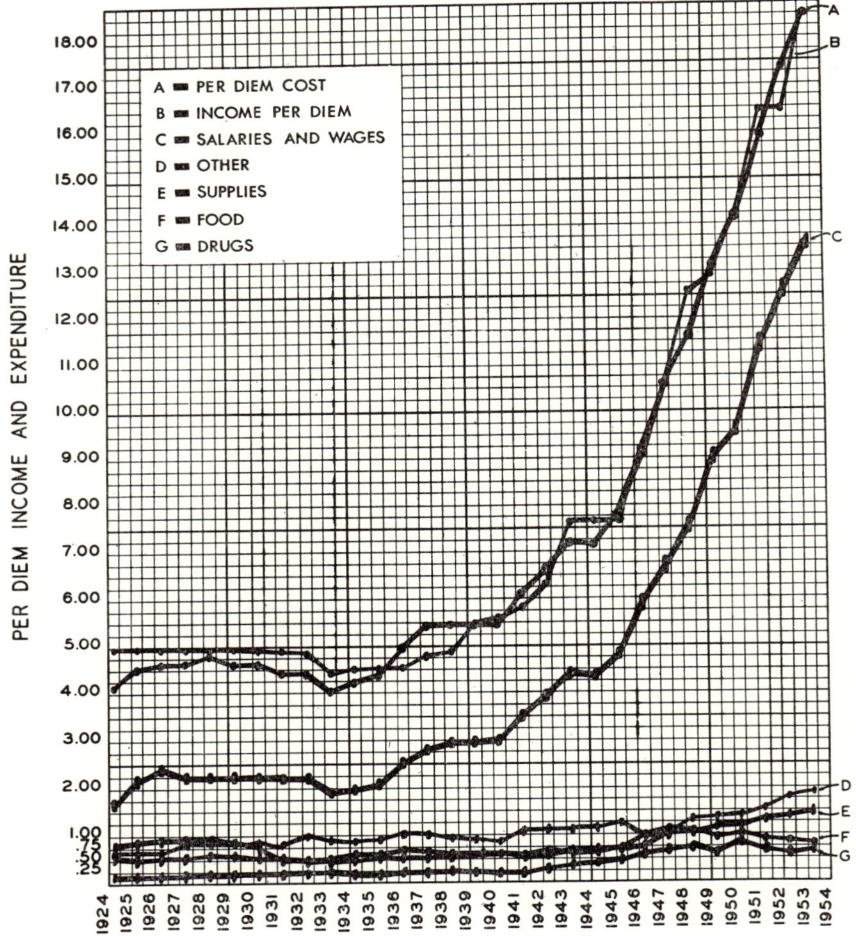

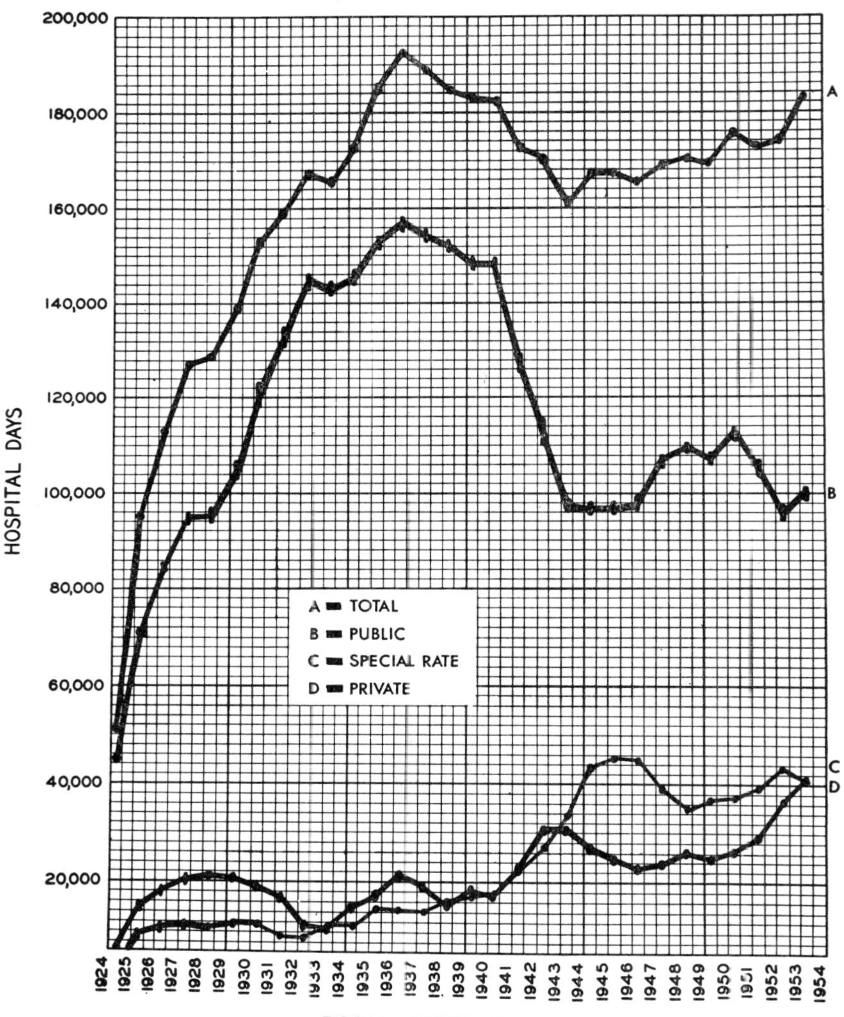
PATIENT DAYS BY CLASSIFICATION
1924-1954
200,000
180,000
160,000
140,000
120,000
100,000
80,000
60,000
40,000
20,000
HOSPITAL DAYS
A TOTAL
B PUBLIC
C SPECIAL RATE
D PRIVATE
A
B
C
D
1924
1925
1926
1927
1928
1929
1930
1931
1932
1933
1934
1935
1936
1937
1938
1939
1940
1941
1942
1943
1944
1945
1946
1947
1948
1949
1950
1951
1952
1953
1954
FISCAL YEARS 1924-1954

expenditure had been $37,697,888.79. The graphs of patient days and per diem income, prepared for the thirtieth anniversary of the hospital in 1954, show well the overall story of service to the state.

Dr. Robin C. Buerki was the first and for almost twenty years the highly efficient superintendent of the Wisconsin General Hospital; he had a drive that enabled him to jump hurdles and he was good at wangling when that was the only way out. Miss Helen Denne, the first head of the hospital nursing staff and director of the new school of nursing, was also involved in the bustling turmoil of those early days. She says: "Dr. Buerki was terrific. He was seemingly on all six floors at once even before the elevators were installed." [3]

Dr. Buerki took his first two years of medical training here at Wisconsin and completed the work for his medical degree at the University of Pennsylvania in 1917. After a period in the army and in private practice, he returned to Wisconsin to take on the involved tasks of getting the new hospital into running order for patients, for the medical and nursing staff, and for medical students. All who were here remember that Buerki's door was always open whatever the complaint, and of course, at the start these were innumerable. Later, he also served as executive secretary of the medical faculty.

Some misunderstanding of the different categories of patients has always existed and has been a cause for grievances. Dr. Buerki, who had been in private practice, was highly appreciative of the difficulties and met the discussions in medical society meetings with understanding.

From 1938 to 1940 at the request of the Commission on Graduate Medical Education, Dr. Buerki was granted leave of absence to direct this study with the aid of a group of first-rate medical educators. The problems of satisfactory internship, hospital residencies, post-graduate education, and specialty boards were carefully considered and presented (1940).[4] During his absence, Dr. William D. Stovall served well as superintendent of the hospital, along with all of his other duties. Buerki returned to Madison in 1940, but a year later was pulled away to become dean of the University of Pennsylvania Graduate School of Medicine and director of the hospitals there.

Following Dr. Buerki's resignation, Dr. Harold M. Coon, who had also taken his first two years of medical training in Wisconsin (1920) and his subsequent work for the M.D. degree (1922) at the University of Pennsylvania, was chosen by Dean Middleton as superintendent. Coon had

had experience in hospital administration as director of the River Pines Sanatorium between 1923 and 1937 and as superintendent at the Wisconsin State Sanatorium between 1937 and 1941. Dr. Coon was prompt in his decisions, a bit peremptory at times; he maintained the attitudes of the physician-superintendent, important arbiter in most of the early hospitals of the country. Such decisions required medical knowledge and judgment as well as a hotel-management type of experience, an increasingly rare combination. The nicety of his housekeeping was one of Dr. Coon's special interests; he visited briefly each ward every day.

You will remember that Dr. Coon was short and fat. You may even remember his familiar nickname. His general form and that of his close friend and classmate, Bob Gilman, who was long and lean, gave Dr. Bunting the opportunity to dub them Mutt and Jeff. Dr. Coon carried on during the difficult World War II period under the leadership of Dr. Walter Meek as acting dean of the Medical School and continued after Dean Middleton's return well beyond the terminal date of this history.

The increasing subdivision of medical practice and the growth of the supporting sciences has made necessary the teaching of technical disciplines that are practiced in hospitals, public health laboratories, and by independent groups of physicians, without requiring the prolonged training needed for the M.D. degree. Four-year courses leading to a bachelor's degree in the respective fields have become available in university medical schools such as Wisconsin and commonly also briefer courses taught in the hospital laboratories, providing a certificate of achievement upon completion of the work. In the Wisconsin General Hospital, both the hospital staff and the medical school faculty have worked together for the common objectives. The well-organized four-year course for medical technicians leading to the B.S. degree has used to advantage the hospital laboratories and the clinical material for the last year of its course of study under Miss Alice Thorngate.

Under Dr. E. A. Pohle, a twelve-month course in X-ray technology has been developed to provide suitably trained personnel for this essential aid in diagnosis. This course does not carry university credit but students receive a certificate following satisfactory completion of the work.

The term "physical medicine" and several related terms will be found in catalogues and dictionaries to confuse the unwary. James Claude

Elsom, M.D., listed in the early catalogues as director of the gymnasium and professor of physical culture, gave some of his time to corrective exercises and may therefore be considered the first person in the University to practice physical therapy. With women students, Helen Dobson Denniston, M.D., carried on similar functions. After the Wisconsin General Hospital and the four-year Medical School became operative, a subdepartment of physical therapy was created under the department of surgery with Dr. Elsom in charge; courses were offered for the third- and fourth-year students and other qualified persons, and physical treatment of different types was made available for patients. Instruction in physical therapy dates from 1927. In 1929, this phase of medicine, still under Dr. Elsom, was placed in the department of radiology under Dr. Ernst A. Pohle. It was further developed by Dr. Frances Hellebrandt, formerly of the department of physiology, and in 1946, the larger field of physical medicine was placed under Dr. Elizabeth Grimm in the department of medicine. After the resignation of Dr. Grimm, physical medicine became a subdepartment of medicine under Dr. Harry D. Bouman. Dr. Bouman had most of his professional training in Holland. When he joined our faculty in 1946 he already had an impressive list of research papers in nerve and muscle physiology to his credit. He continued his productive career and also advanced the field by becoming the competent editor of the *American Journal of Physical Medicine*.[5]

Physical therapy has for some years been in the effective hands of Miss Margaret Kohli. In 1945, a four-year course leading to the B.S. degree and a certificate in physical therapy was offered.

Occupational therapy was started in 1926 in the hospital under the direction of Miss Frances T. Stuart; she continued as supervisor and instructor until her retirement in 1949. Both Dr. Frances Hellebrandt and Dr. Elizabeth Grimm gave further impetus to this mode of therapy. In 1945, Dr. Grimm was succeeded by Miss Caroline G. Thompson, who has carried on this work well beyond our historical period. In 1943 occupational therapy was accepted as a four-year course, with the privilege of granting a B.S. degree.

The main functions of the hospital are manifest; the details are so multitudinous with both homely and professional services to thousands of patients that a history of many pages would be required to tell the story adequately. In this synoptic history only a few of the special services can be mentioned.

A proper diet is a demanding need of those who are ill. As Owen Meredith has facetiously put it:

> We may live without friends; we may live without books;
> But civilized man cannot live without cooks.

The culinary arts and details, such as specific weighed diets in diseases like diabetes, are among the essential services of a hospital.

Miss Viola Maag served as chief dietitian from April, 1923, to July, 1927. She assisted Dr. Elmer Sevringhaus in writing *Instructions for Diabetic Patients in Wisconsin General Hospital*, first published in 1924. Instructions and diets for persons suffering from diabetes and also reducing diets were included in the first publication. In the eleventh edition, 1942, other frequently used hospital diets were included and the name changed to *Dietetic Manual*.

The immaculate kitchen where the food is prepared, the preheated stainless steel trucks to keep the food hot while in transit to all the wards, and the trays for the patients served directly from the diet kitchen in each ward are prepared in accordance with the orders of the physician. Since 1942, this complex organization has been under the efficient care of Miss Ruth Dickie.

In addition to serving thousands of meals daily, the dietary department conducts extensive educational programs. Patients are instructed in the proper food they should eat after leaving the hospital whenever there is a special dietary problem associated with their illness.

The dispensing of drugs is another important part of the story of the hospital. The striking changes in medical practice may be observed in a nutshell by studying the changes in the prescriptions the pharmacist filled during the first quarter-century of the hospital.

Osler's battle against one of the misuses of drugs merits a quotation.

The battle against poly-pharmacy, or the use of a large number of drugs (of the action of which we know little, yet we put them into bodies of the action of which we know less), has not been fought to a finish. . . . A new school of practitioners has arisen which cares nothing for homoeopathy and less for so-called allopathy. It seeks to study, rationally and scientifically, the action of drugs, old and new. It is more concerned that a physician shall know how to apply the few great medicines which all have to use, such as quinine, iron, mercury, iodide of potassium, opium and digitalis, than that he should employ a multiplicity of remedies the action of which is extremely doubtful.[6]

The Wisconsin General Hospital did not open its doors until years after many of the worst of the mixtures were discarded. The bacteriologic revolution was in full swing, and Behring and Kitasato had introduced the serum therapy period by the use of diphtheria and tetanus antitoxin (Nobel Prize, 1901). This era tended to persist until reasonably effective active immunization made passive immunity against these diseases less needed. Other Nobel Prizes have been awarded to honor those who by their discoveries have greatly increased therapeutic measures. Immediately one thinks of specific chemotherapy and #606 — salvarsan of Ehrlich and Hata, 1907 (Nobel Prize in 1927) and other arsenicals. Later Prontosil (Domagk), sulfanilamide, and the many sulfa drugs were added. The glandular substitution therapy, such as insulin for diabetes (Banting and Macleod, Nobel Prize, 1923) and liver therapy in treatment of pernicious anemia (Whipple, Minot, and Murphy; Nobel Prize, 1934), gave another valuable type of prescription to the pharmacist. The introduction of penicillin during World War II was the beginning of a long list of potent antibiotics.

The hospital pharmacy does not have the colorful blue and red globes and stunning ceramic pots inscribed with the names of ancient drugs as did the corner drugstore of seventy years ago, nor the penny stick of peppermint and wintergreen candy, nor that indescribable aroma. But the druggist or pharmacist — in or out of the hospital — has always aimed at accuracy. "Always check the label on the bottle when you take it off the shelf and again when you put it back" is one of their precepts. Mr. Ernst Kuenzi was our first and long-time pharmacist, who gave excellent service and trained good men to follow him. We salute them all.

26 The School of Nursing and Nursing Services in the University of Wisconsin

Nursing, as an art to be cultivated, as a profession to be followed, is modern; nursing, as a practice, originated in the dim past when some mother among the cave dwellers cooled the forehead of her sick child with water from the brook or first yielded to the prompting to leave a well-covered bone or a handful of meal by the side of a wounded man left in the hurried flight before an enemy. A luxury let us say in her private capacity, in public, the trained nurse has become one of the great blessings of humanity taking a place beside the physician and the priest and not inferior to either in her mission.
William Osler

Nurses and the members of the nursing profession hold a high place in the minds and hearts of those to whom they have ministered, on the field of battle, in the hospital, or in the home. But that has not always been so. We immediately think of the drunken Mrs. Sairey Gamp of Dickens' *Martin Chuzzlewit*, or by way of sharp contrast, the mission of Florence Nightingale during the Crimean War and later, and in our country, Dorothea L. Dix, crusading for care of patients in hospitals for the insane and acting as superintendent of women nurses during our Civil War.

Just as medical schools in Britain developed in and around hospitals, so in this country and in Canada schools of nursing grew up in hospitals because of the manifest needs. Gradually the better hospitals, especially those affiliated with medical schools, improved the instruction with increasing emphasis on the underlying sciences as well as the art of nursing. The Flexner reports (1910–12) on medical education in the United States and Canada and in Europe greatly accelerated the advances in medical

203

education, so that the changes were almost revolutionary. Similarly, but to a lesser extent, the report of the committee for the study of nursing education with C.-E. A. Winslow, professor of public health at Yale, as chairman, and Josephine Goldmark, as secretary, was of the utmost importance. This scholarly report (1923) came as a result of the conference called by the Rockefeller Foundation in 1918 to consider the development of public health nursing in the United States. The conference also considered the problems of nurses on private duty, the training of the nurse in hospital schools, and urged "the development and strengthening of university schools of nursing as of fundamental importance."[1] Postgraduate courses, especially for public health nursing, were stressed. Following the publication of the Goldmark report, three private university schools of nursing in the United States and Canada were endowed by the Rockefeller Foundation, and one by Mrs. Frances Paine Bolton of Cleveland, Ohio.

Nursing education and service in Wisconsin developed along with the growth of the state and the country. In 1920, there were forty-two hospital diploma schools in Wisconsin. In the University of Wisconsin an effort to start a School of Nursing was made soon after the Bradley Hospital and the Student Infirmary were completed. Miss Florence Patterson came here from the Johns Hopkins Hospital school to initiate a three-year diploma program. This did not flourish; the facilities were inadequate to meet the requisite standards. Within a few years, the school was closed, the students were transferred to hospital schools elsewhere, and Miss Patterson resigned.

The completion of the Wisconsin General Hospital gave a second opportunity for the University to establish a School of Nursing. The legislative act providing funds for the construction of the hospital also gave moneys specifically for the building of a nurses' dormitory, thus emphasizing the importance of the nursing function.

Accordingly Drs. Bardeen and Evans had conferences in medical schools and schools for nurses in several parts of the country. In Chicago, Dr. E. E. Irons of Rush Medical College and Presbyterian Hospital proved most helpful. He recommended Miss Helen Denne, a young supervisor at Presbyterian Hospital and a graduate of Queens University in Kingston, Ontario; she was offered the post. The suggested position was a heavy challenge, combining the tasks of director of the School of Nursing and superintendent of the nursing services of the hospital. The urging of Dr.

Irons and other Chicago friends of our school, visits to Madison, and further contacts with Dr. Evans at his persuasive best and with President Birge, whom she called "the grandest man," finally resulted in a telegram of acceptance.

Miss Denne was a crusader; she insisted that a university school of nursing should be an integral part of the institution and be accepted as such. President Birge said, "You will have to go slow. There is no money. You will have to persuade the parents of the girls that there is good value in your offerings and you will have to persuade the faculty that the course merits university credit and support." Miss Denne gained the attention, the respect and then the support of the leaders of the faculty, and finally the necessary vote.

Dean Sellery's support was most helpful and essential. He and his faculty agreed that the proposed School of Nursing could be under the College of Letters and Science and the students could register in that college provided they fulfilled the requirements of the college. This became the important basis for the inception and growth of the School of Nursing.

Miss Denne took over her manifold and exciting tasks in 1924 with Dr. Robin C. Buerki as the energetic, exuberant superintendent of the hospital. She stated: "We started before we were ready to start, but we started. We purchased everything. We opened a new house for the nurses every day by a rapid transformation of the former private residences." [2]

The School of Nursing was organized in association with the Medical School of the University and with the Wisconsin General Hospital. The admission requirements were those of the University. Originally, two courses were offered. A three-year course leading to the certificate of graduate nurse required at least one semester of academic work and thirty-two months of professional training in residence in the School of Nursing. The other course included a combination of five years of study leading to the R.N. certificate and the Bachelor of Science degree, either in the College of Letters and Science or the College of Agriculture, depending on the academic course chosen.

Miss Denne was the leader. She was not tall, but her posture, dignity, and assurance gave one the impression of a commanding personality. She was a dominant person; she needed all her persistence in the establishment of the school. After the nurses' dormitory was completed in 1926 and the Nursing School had become a more complete unit, she interested herself in all the details of the lives of the girls, such as a separate dining room and the necessary resources for a gracious, comfortable environment. She and her staff with the help of **Dr. Bardeen, Dr. Buerki,** and other members of the Medical School faculty succeeded in building up an *esprit de corps* among the student nurses, a sense of belonging to an institution of importance and one that cared for each individual. While the student nurses were in residence in the hospital, tuition was remitted and room and board were provided in the dormitory as an appropriate return for care of the patients.

An important difference in the practice of this school as compared with many others was that the educational opportunities for the student nurses were always the central focus of the school. A registered nurse was in charge on the wards, and even though responsibilities were given increasingly to the student nurses as they advanced in their course, a supervisor-instructor was always available.

Miss Lila B. Fletcher joined Miss Denne immediately in 1924 as second-in-command in the nursing service, a position she held until the functions of the Nursing School and the nursing services were separated at the time of Miss Denne's resignation in 1937. At that time, Miss Christina Murray was appointed Director of the School of Nursing, and Miss Fletcher became Superintendent of Nursing Services. Miss Fletcher was also a graduate of the Presbyterian Hospital School of Nursing and had been a close friend of Miss Denne as they served on the staff of that hospital. She supplemented Miss Denne exceptionally well. Smiling, serene, with a quiet voice, she seemed to say, "No need for excitement; everything will come out all right." At the same time she maintained high standards, had a delightful sense of humor, and an innate gaiety of approach to life. She was a good administrator, objective and fair-minded. During the latter years of Miss Fletcher's service, Miss Marjorie Paquin, one of the early collegiate graduates of the school, became an especially strong supervisor and aid. Following Miss Fletcher's death, Miss Paquin became Superintendent of Nursing Services.

Miss Christina C. Murray served as full-time instructor in the Wisconsin School of Nursing from 1925 to 1930, when she went to England for study on an exchange scholarship. After teaching in several Canadian schools she returned to Wisconsin in 1937 as the second Director of the School of Nursing (1937–48). She was a graduate of the University of Saskatchewan and of the Royal Victoria Hospital School of Nursing in Montreal. She was a model of precise nicety for her students. Her turns of speech, her demonstrations in the class room and at the bedside, relieved by a sense of humor, are recalled with pleasure by her students and her colleagues. Her natural grace was shown also when, in a black velvet costume trimmed with white fur, she drew beautiful skating figures on the ice.

Miss Margery MacLachlan (1900–63) was the first graduate of Wisconsin's School of Nursing, having earned in 1927 the degree of B.S. and the certificate of graduate nurse. After broad experience in teaching in a number of hospital schools in widely different geographical areas and at Yale University School of Nursing, she returned to Wisconsin as the third Director of the School of Nursing at the end of our period in 1949.

The students of the first class of the School of Nursing entered the University in the fall of 1924, and in February, 1925, began their hospital residence and training. Twelve received their certificates of Graduate Nurse in June, 1927, including two who also earned their B.S. degrees. The School grew steadily, and in 1950, fifty-nine young women earned the nursing R.N. certificate; of these, thirty also qualified for the B.S. degree. The School of Nursing used as its major clinical field the State of Wisconsin General Hospital. However, other hospitals and agencies in Madison, Milwaukee, and other cities have assisted in the teaching program. For example, for a number of years the Chicago Lying-In Hospital and Dispensary served as the clinical field for obstetrics and for all students in the School of Nursing. This was also true for the medical students during the early years.

The curriculum of the School of Nursing has followed the changes in medical practice and the increasing affluence of the country; public health nursing has been added and also special work in ward management. Details are far too involved to present in this history which is intended chiefly to give some idea of the men and women who have given their devotion to the schools. A relationship of mutual appreciation has existed between the medical and nursing schools; many of the members of the Medical School faculty have provided courses for the student nurses. The regular faculty of the School of Nursing has enjoyed the same tenure privileges as have the Regent appointees in other divisions of the University. The nursing service staff, frequently the same persons, have also enjoyed similar privileges and relationships.

Not only in our School of Nursing but elsewhere, nurses have commonly been too busy ministering to their patients to write much about their duties or their efforts to improve the services. By stretching our time limits slightly I am able to include a commendable publication from our nursing group. During his long Johns Hopkins period, Dr. John Harris stimulated Carolyn C. Van Blarcom to write a successful book on obstetrical nursing that passed through three editions — 1922, 1928, and 1933. By the time Dr. Harris came to Wisconsin, Miss Van Blarcom was unable to write the necessary revision, and Miss Erna Ziegel, supervisor of our obstetrical and gynecological services was persuaded by Dr. Harris to take over this task. Beginning in the early 1940's, she spent more than ten years on this effort. The fourth revised edition by Miss Ziegel has had distinct success and is an example of Dr. Harris' splendid influence.[3]

Through the twenty-five years of this history, the School of Nursing and the nursing services in the hospitals have been fortunate in the high qualifications of their leaders and in the support accorded by the faculties of the University. Miss Denne stated that one serious hazard in the continuity of nursing, a difficulty which she herself was unable to evade, is matrimony. After observing the girls on the wards and in the classroom and chatting with them, I am entirely persuaded that that hazard is unavoidable.

27 Cancer Research

It is far better that occult cancers were left untreated; for those who are treated readily expire; whereas those who are not treated may endure a long time.

Hippocrates

American physicians and scientists began to organize their attack on cancer about the beginning of the twentieth century, and by 1928 the Wisconsin cancer program was making progress under the leadership of Dr. W. D. Stovall. Quite early, the study of malignant growth, such as crown gall in plants, was begun in the department of plant pathology with Joyce Riker as chief of investigation. In the 1920's, M. F. Guyer of the department of zoology was studying transplantable tumors in mice and certain hereditary eye defects in rabbits in collaboration with Frederick A. Davis of our Medical School staff.

Cancer research received a major lift in 1934 by a bequest of approximately $420,000 in the will of Miss Jenny Bowman in memory of her father, Jonathan Bowman. The will provided that the money should be used for fundamental studies regarding the nature and cure of cancer. The administration of the fund was placed in the hands of Dr. Charles R. Bardeen, then dean of the Medical School. A committee consisting of Drs. Bardeen, W. J. Meek, chairman of the department of physiology, and Gunnar Gundersen, prominent alumnus, member of the University Board of Regents, and practicing physician from La Crosse, was authorized to visit leading centers of tumor research and to make recommendations. In their report to President Frank, we can see Bardeen's guiding hand urging the selection of several younger men of promise, giving them opportunity, fellowships, or money for travel study rather than putting all the eggs in one basket, hoping to find one prominent ideal man.

Accordingly, in 1935, three fellows were selected — Drs. Harold P. Rusch in physiology, Fred Mohs in zoology, and Mead Burke in pathology. Highly interesting is the fact that both Rusch and Mohs went on to devote their lives to work in tumor studies. Dr. Mohs' work in chemosurgery has become an integral part of the department of surgery and has been presented more fully in the chapter on that department.

Under the auspices of the Wisconsin Alumni Research Foundation, a Cancer Institute was held here at the Medical School in September, 1936; many leading cancer specialists took part, including three from foreign countries. Lectures, conferences, and discussions covered many aspects of the field including genetics, diagnostic problems, the early recognition of malignant tumors, X-ray therapy, filterable viruses, tissue culture, cytology, and etiology. The meetings provided a broad basis for the planning of future cancer research.

A second gift of high importance came in May, 1935 — a bequest of Michael McArdle of Baileys Harbor, Wisconsin, for the promotion of cancer studies here at the University. Because of meager space, Dean Middleton urged that a new building be erected for all cancer research conducted within the Medical School. This plan was approved and an excellent four-story building was constructed with McArdle funds ($132,000) and additional aid of $108,000 from a Public Works Administration grant. The McArdle memorial laboratory, first occupied in March, 1940, provided the hoped-for opportunities. Support for the research at this laboratory came chiefly from two sources — the interest from the Bowman funds, which amounted to between $11,000 and $12,000 annually, and a direct yearly appropriation of $10,000 from the State of Wisconsin. Smaller grants have been obtained from other sources.[1]

Obviously the men involved in such studies are more significant than the physical plant, despite the importance of adequate space and equipment. Cancer research has been fortunate in both respects. From the time of his appointment in 1935, the smilingly confident Dr. Rusch has continued his progress as an investigator in the cancer field and as head of the McArdle Laboratory after its completion in 1940. He has shown that best of all attributes in an administrator — good judgment in the choice of his associates. An informal cooperative spirit of investigation has pervaded the well-organized laboratory.

Dr. Rusch, a native of Wisconsin, took his undergraduate work and also his medical studies here at Wisconsin, receiving the M.D. degree in

1933. He continued his training in Wisconsin General Hospital as an intern and then enjoyed a series of fellowships leading to the directorship of the McArdle Laboratory.

Only a representative few of the significant advances made in the laboratories during the first decade of its history can be cited. The carcinogenic properties of ultraviolet irradiation were located between 2900 and 3341 angstroms, the most potent wave length in the production of erythema.[2] In studies on the influence of diet, greater caloric intake, especially of fat, increased the rate of tumor formation in certain albino mice.[3] In studying chemical carcinogens, the influence of dietary pyridoxine and casein on the carcinogenicity of p-dimethylaminoazobenzene showed that the number of hepatomas in rats fed on synthetic diets was influenced by their nutritional history.[4]

Dr. Van R. Potter, biochemist, philosopher, and enthusiast, joined the McArdle staff in 1940, and later became assistant director. His early training had been in South Dakota State College and in the department of biochemistry at Wisconsin (Ph.D., 1938). Potter and his associates have devoted their attention to complex enzyme systems in normal and tumor tissues through the study of tissue slices and minces and by isolated enzyme techniques. They have advanced our knowledge of aerobic glycolysis, the type of metabolism characteristic of tumor tissue, and have studied the mechanism of hydrogen transport in animal tissues.[5] They have found also that the cytochrome c content of several experimental tumors is less than in normal tissues, thus lending further support to Warburg's idea that tumor tissue is better able to withstand anaerobic conditions than is normal tissue.[6]

The only other members of the increasing McArdle staff who come within our time spectrum are Drs. James A. and Elizabeth C. Miller. James Miller did his undergraduate work at the University of Pittsburgh and his graduate training here at the University of Wisconsin in biochemistry, obtaining his Ph.D. degree in 1943. Both Miller and his wife Elizabeth (Ph.D. Wisconsin, 1945), have been eager, meticulous collaborators in a fine series of studies on the influence of certain dyes on carcinogenesis.[7]

The post–World War II period with its explosive developments in many areas gave large funds and opportunities to the McArdle cancer group. Many appointments followed, but both the men and their research must await another chronicler.

Although the McArdle faculty does not teach any regular medical students as did their colleagues in the earlier Wisconsin Psychiatric Institute, nonetheless they began almost immediately to have graduate students even before that privilege was accorded them by the graduate school faculty. Four men, Kenneth P. DuBois, James A. Bain, James M. Price, and Gerald C. Mueller, who received their Ph.D. degrees officially with majors in physiology, actually did their research with men of the oncology group. Since then, the various training programs in the McArdle laboratories have increased astoundingly, so that the faculty members do have teaching responsibilities on a productive scholarship level.

Queries have arisen as to the proper position and use of research institutes in our American universities and more specifically here in the University of Wisconsin. The greater autonomy, the exceptional research opportunities in this "publish or perish" era, more technical aids and larger sums of money, as well as the lack of contact with any but graduate students are factors that need consideration. It seems probable that such specifically oriented institutes will increase. How then may they best be woven into the fabric and life of the schools and colleges of the University?

28 World War II

After Hitler and the German army overran Poland in 1939, Britain and France declared war. Shortly thereafter the *Blitzkrieg* conquered Holland, Belgium, and France. The day Paris fell, June 14, 1940, and the thrilling rescue of the British Expeditionary Force from the beaches of Dunkirk are indelible in our memories. Britain stood alone under her indomitable leader, Churchill. Inevitably, as in World War I, the United States was drawn into the maelstrom. The re-elected President Roosevelt promised all aid short of war. We traded destroyers to Britain in return for naval bases and initiated the Lend-Lease program. Ruthless submarine warfare on the part of Germany against our ships and the destruction of our Pacific fleet by Japan at Pearl Harbor on December 7, 1941, brought America overwhelmingly into the war. The University of Wisconsin under President Dykstra carried on a military-civilian schedule similar to that in World War I, stressing our obligation to be a training ground for the armed forces as well as an institution committed to civilian education. Most of the medical students and many of the faculty were required to continue their regular training and teaching duties on a three-semester schedule. In his 1942–44 report to the Regents, President Dykstra stated that in the last three years the University had given special training to more than 12,000 men and women for the armed forces.

Many of our men, both faculty and alumni, performed heroic service in all the theaters of war.

The 135th medical regiment, first under the command of Col. William J. Bleckwenn and later under Col. Marc J. Musser, both of the University, was a front-line unit operating with the American Sixth Army, which took part in most of the heavy invasions from Buna through the liberation of the Phillipine Islands.

A National Guard unit, the 135th, secured its enlisted personnel from Wisconsin and its staff of doctors from the Wisconsin General hospital, the University, Marquette University, and Wisconsin physicians. The 44th, on the other hand, was commanded by Col. Frank L. Weston, chief of medicine, Col. Joseph W. Gale, chief of surgery, and Ida Bechtold, chief nurse, all University personnel. Nurses for the 44th came from Wisconsin and adjoining states, and in some instances medical students from the University were taken into the corps as they neared graduation.

A general hospital unit, the 44th was equipped to handle any kind of emergency; the seriously wounded were immediately sent back to one of the units of the 44th. While the 135th was a frontline casualty outfit, both Wisconsin units saw combat action, and each had encounters with attacking Japanese forces.

"Portions of our unit, which went overseas in March, 1942, established the first American field hospital in the Southwest Pacific theater," related Col. Musser. "It was located . . . near Darwin, and operated in support of Australian and American troops responsible for the defense of the Northern Australian coast against an anticipated Japanese invasion. Another operated the first hospital in New Guinea during the Buna campaign, caring for casualties from the 32nd division."

In early 1943, following the Buna campaign, the regiment built and operated a 1,000-bed hospital at Port Moresby [New Guinea] which was the largest and most complete American hospital north of Australia at that time.

The ability of the 135th to build hospitals, despite material shortages and lack of engineers, soon brought it the nickname, known throughout the theater, of "The 135th Medical Engineers."

"The unit operated its own sawmill and did all of its own construction," Musser grinned.

During the remainder of 1943 and 1944 medical units were provided by the regiment, which was redesignated the 135th medical group in 1944.

.   .   .   .

But the 135th was not alone in encountering Japanese forces. In spite of its more secure position at the base of the medical echelon, the 44th hospital corps also ran into considerable combat action.

Though commissioned much earlier, the 44th had been activated in January, 1943, and after nine months of training at Fort Sill, Oklahoma, was transported to Australia.

"After a period of staging," Col. Weston, chief of medicine, explained, "it was planned that we should function in Milne Bay. But our ship hit a reef, and we were forced into a change of plans."

After setting up hospitals and operating in Queensland, Australia, until

October, 1944, the group was scheduled for participation in the Leyte campaign.

"We . . . landed on Leyte Nov. 18, setting up a hospital at Buraun," Col. Weston said. "We began operation in tents Dec. 5, and after six months in this area we moved to a more desirable and more complete installation on the beach.

"The six months in Leyte our group was actually on the front line — far in advance of where a general hospital is supposed to be," he added. "We were mixed up in some Japanese paratroop action from Dec. 6 until the 10th, and were directly attacked by Japs the night of Dec. 10. . . ."

"It was a little rough," Weston smiled. "We had our own perimeter, and were well armed — contrary to all the laws of war, but necessary because of the enemy attitude toward hospitals.

"They were repulsed, however," he said, "and we had only two casualties; Edward Birge, then a major, grandson of the president emeritus of the University, and James Bingham, then a captain."

During the period on Leyte the 44th general hospital was taking casualties directly from the front line as well as evacuation casualties from other islands.[1]

The service records of the faculty of the University of Wisconsin Medical School as well as of physicians throughout the state are much more complete than for World War I. This is due in considerable part to the excellent memorial, *War Without Guns* (1949), published by the State Medical Society of Wisconsin. This book presents a biographical sketch of most of the Wisconsin physicians who served in World War II during the period from Pearl Harbor, December 7, 1941, to V. J. Day, August 14, 1945. The rosters of the Wisconsin Group Practice Units — the 44th Hospital Unit, the 32nd Division Medical Units, and the 135th Medical Regiment — are presented with appropriate prominence. Although these units were drawn from the whole state of Wisconsin, members of our faculty and also alumni practicing in different areas of the state are included; I am therefore using these rosters as a means of presenting briefly the many Wisconsin physicians who gave major service in World War II.[2]

ROSTER OF THE 44th HOSPITAL UNIT

Maj. Abner P. Bennett, Evansville, Indiana

Lt. Col. John E. Bentley, Madison

Lt. Col. Edward A. Birge, Milwaukee

Lt. Col. Einar R. Daniels, Milwaukee

Maj. William Esser, Sheboygan

Lt. Col. Richard W. Farnsworth, Janesville

Col. Joseph W. Gale, Madison
Maj. Chester Gjertson, Madison
Lt. Col. Edgar S. Gordon, Madison
Lt. Col. A. A. Holbrook, Milwaukee
Maj. Homer H. Kohler, Sheboygan
Maj. Roy B. Larsen, Wausau
Lt. Col. K. E. Lemmer, Madison
Capt. Bertrand W. Meyer, Madison
Lt. Col. Peter A. Midelfart, Eau Claire
Capt. Myron A. Meyers, Bloomington
Lt. Col. Jerry W. McRoberts, Sheboygan
Lt. Col. Joseph Pessin, Burbank, California
Maj. H. W. Pohle, Milwaukee
Maj. Jackman Pyre, Tuscon, Arizona
Maj. S. C. Rogers, Madison
Maj. Edward G. Schott, Sheboygan
Lt. Col. H. H. Shapiro, Madison
Maj. J. L. Sims, Madison
Capt. H. J. Tausend, Madison
Lt. Col. F. D. Weeks, Ashland
Col. F. L. Weston, Madison, C. O.
Col. Edward F. Westover, Madison

ROSTER OF THE 32nd DIVISION MEDICAL UNITS

Col. William Bleckwenn, Madison
Col. G. J. Hathaway, Superior
Col. Marc J. Musser, Madison
Lt. Col. Reinhard Becker, West Allis
Lt. Col. Walter T. Becker, Wausau
Lt. Col. Eben Carey, Milwaukee
Lt. Col. L. S. Eagleburger, Waupun
Lt. Col. Harry Heiden, Sheboygan
Lt. Col. Fred G. Hidde, Sheboygan
Lt. Col. Stanley W. Hollenbeck, Milwaukee
Lt. Col. Edward H. Leveroos, Superior
Lt. Col. James E. Miller, Madison
Lt. Col. Carl Nebel, Milwaukee
Lt. Col. Louis W. Nowack, Watertown

Lt. Col. Leo W. Peterson, Sun Prairie
Lt. Col. Fred J. Pohle, Madison
Lt. Col. Lester L. Weissmiller, Madison
Lt. Col. Sylvester S. Zintek, Milwaukee
Maj. Leo M. Boxer, Racine
Maj. James W. Brooke, Madison
Maj. Wilmer H. Christiansen, Milwaukee
Maj. James W. Ferris, Milwaukee
Maj. John A. Gallogly, Milwaukee
Lt. Col. John Grab, Sun Prairie
Maj. Robert S. Haukohl, Milwaukee
Maj. Clement J. Moran, Hines, Ill.
Maj. Richard E. Muenzner, Milwaukee
Maj. John O'D. McCabe, Wauwatosa
Maj. M. J. Schramel, Milwaukee
Maj. Herbert B. Shields, Milwaukee
Maj. Philip M. Wilkinson, Oconomowoc
Capt. Herbert B. Christianson, Superior
Capt. Chalmer Davee, River Falls
Capt. Bernard T. Fein, Milwaukee
Capt. John F. Holmes, Milton Junction
Capt. Thurman E. Kendall, Milwaukee
Capt. Raymond K. McMahon, Madison
Capt. Cyril A. Schwarz, Watertown
Capt. John N. Thanos, Milwaukee
Capt. Edward W. Vetter, Fond du Lac

ROSTER OF THE 135th MEDICAL REGIMENT

Lt. Duane Alexander, MAC, Madison
Lt. Col. Ed Bachhuber, MC, Milwaukee
Col. Reinhard Becker, MC, Milwaukee
Col. Walter T. Becker, MC, Wausau
Lt. Stanford Benner, MAC, Madison
Col. William Bleckwenn, MC, Madison
Lt. Col. Leo M. Boxer, MC, Racine
W. O. Charles L. Braem, Marshfield
Lt. Thomas Carroll, MAC, Wauwatosa
Maj. Wilmer Christiansen, MC, Milwaukee

Capt. Emil De Amann, MAC, Milwaukee
Lt. Leon Dorsch, MAC, Soldiers Grove
Col. Leon S. Eagleburger, MC, Waupun
Capt. Dana W. Foss, DC, Hudson
Maj. Lawrence W. Gabert, DC, Milwaukee
Capt. Anthony J. Gagliano, MAC, Milwaukee
Maj. John A. Gallogly, MC, Milwauke
Lt. Col. Robert S. Haukohl, MC, Milwaukee
Maj. Albert G. Hemer (Chaplain), Mondovi
Capt. Ray J. Heuck, MAC, Milwaukee
Col. Fred G. Hidde, MC, Sheboygan
Maj. John F. Holmes, MC, Milton Junction
Capt. Elmer P. Huth, MC, Wauwatosa
Lt. Col. Anselm M. Keefe (Chaplain), West De Pere
Maj. Thurman E. Kendall, MC, Racine
Capt. Ray F. Kuhlman, MC, Milwaukee
Capt. Elmer Lipinski, MC, Milwaukee
Capt. Robert V. Lloyd, MAC, Appleton
Lt. John J. Looze, MAC, Madison
Col. Erwin P. Ludwig, MC, Wausau
Maj. John O'D. McCabe, MC, Milwaukee
Maj. Ray McMahon, MC, Madison
Maj. James H. Mackin, MAC, Madison
Maj. Joe M. Mano, FC, Madison
Maj. Robert O. Meng, DC, Madison
Maj. William F. Metzler, DC, Milwaukee
Lt. Col. James E. Miller, MC, Madison
Maj. Frederick Mott, MAC, Madison
Col. Marc J. Musser, MC, Madison
Maj. Michael S. Nefchez, MC, Milwaukee
Maj. Leo P. Perssion, MC, Winnebago
Maj. John R. Peterson, MC, Milwaukee
Col. Leo W. Peterson, MC, Sun Prairie
CWO Maynard Peterson, Marshfield
Capt. Earl Raab, TC, Loyal
Maj. Albert Rasmussen, MAC, Marshfield
Maj. Michael Richdorf, DC, Sheboygan
Capt. Cyril Schwarze, MC, Madison

Maj. John N. Thanos, MC, Milwaukee
Capt. George Theurer, MC, Madison
Maj. George E. Tinkham, DC, Baraboo
Maj. Edward W. Vetter, MC, Fond du Lac
Maj. Don Westra, MAC, Waupun
Lt. Col. Phil M. Wilkinson, MC, Oconomowoc

When Dean Middleton left for war service with the U. S. Medical Corps in Europe in 1942, Dr. Walter J. Meek was appointed acting dean of the Medical School. Despite the many difficulties caused by the war and the personnel problems that are always with us, Dr. Meek strove to uphold the principle of excellence.

Medical faculty listed in the catalogues as on leave for military service are given below; the arrangement is solely on an alphabetical basis. As in the chapter on World War I, I am giving only the names of persons who were members of the medical faculty at the time of their service.

John E. Bentley
James B. Bingham
Edward A. Birge, Jr.
William J. Bleckwenn
Albert J. Borer
James Dollard
Silas M. Evans
Joseph W. Gale
Frederick D. Geist
Edgar S. Gordon
Marvin F. Greiber
Otto V. Hibma
Frank L. Kozelka
Kenneth E. Lemmer
William S. Middleton
Marc J. Musser
Joseph Pessin
Frederick J. Pohle
Hans H. Reese
Charles V. Seastone

Herman H. Shapiro
John B. Wear, Sr.
Lester L. Weissmiller
Frank L. Weston
Edwin F. Westover

After World War II was over, those who had served in the armed forces of the country and those who had served in other capacities began to reshape their lives. On March 1, 1946, a Homecoming Convocation was held by the Medical School to honor the faculty and staff members who served in the armed forces. On May 8, 1946, the University commemorated with deep gratitude the sacrifices of the men and women who "gave their last full measure of devotion" to their country in World War II. Through all the thoughtful addresses and in the minds of each person echoed the humble words of Abraham Lincoln in dedicating the national cemetery at Gettysburg. Another and living memorial to those who fought in World War II stands on our campus — the splendid Memorial Library of the University of Wisconsin, the cornerstone of which was laid in 1950.[3]

29 Buildings and Budgets

*A state so generous in appropriating funds to aid animal
industry could well contribute to the health of its people.*
Governor Emanuel L. Philipp (1920)

The humble beginnings and slow growth, the enthusi-
astic, competent faculty, and the close contacts between students and
faculty of the young Medical School have been considered earlier in this
history. Except for the excellent Student Health Service, the preclinical
branches had a start of almost two decades over the clinical departments,
and both faculty and students established a fine reputation among the
medical schools of the country. The graduates with the B.S. or B.A. degree from Wisconsin including the first two years of medicine were cheerfully accepted by the best of these schools. These students have, to our
delight, commonly retained a deep allegiance to Wisconsin.

The laboratories of the preclinical departments were from the beginning and for years in the upper stories of the old Chemical Engineering
Building at 600 North Park Street and in the top of Science Hall After
the construction of Sterling Hall in 1917, the physics department, which
had been occupying the lower floors of Science Hall, moved to its new
quarters there, and the considerable space they had used was assigned
to the Medical School. The several departments worked happily and successfully there in Science Hall for more than a decade.

The first building occupied by the Student Health Service (1910–11)
was the Cornelius house, a small wooden structure with some mid-Vic-
torian charm, just east of the stone administration building on the corner
of State and Park streets. Now both of these buildings are gone. The
growth of the health service occasioned the acquisition and remodeling
of the Olin house in 1912 and of the Raymer house next door in 1915,

221

both on Langdon Street just east of the President's house, which was then on the corner of N. Park and Langdon streets. A brick addition in the rear of the Raymer house served as a small student infirmary until the present infirmary was completed in 1919–20; offices, X-ray facilities, and the clinical laboratories were developed on the ground floor of the old building. Later these houses, the President's house, and the next one to the east owned by Dean (later President) Birge were razed to provide a suitable site for the Memorial Union.

Members of the faculty and students who have joined the Medical School family since the early 1920's will find it almost impossible to appreciate the excitement and elation of those who were immediately concerned when, in 1916–17, the plans for the Bradley Memorial Hospital and the Student Infirmary were approved. These were the first buildings erected specifically for clinical purposes; they scattered the clouds of doubt that a medical school could ever be developed here.

A careful study was made by Dr. Bardeen and committees both of the faculty and the Regents on the choice of a site for these two buildings. The Langdon Street location had been ruled out as important for broader University functions, and the block facing the Extension and Home Economics Building provided more space centrally located. Bardeen wrote to Van Hise, "We believe that the Regents should look forward definitely to the utilization of the land between the present Physics and Chemistry buildings on the east and the Agricultural Building and University High School on the west as a site for the medical school in its ultimate development." [1]

These two buildings were completed in 1919 and made possible further growth in clinical fields. Dermatology and orthopedic and plastic surgery, under Drs. Foerster, Gaenslen, and Brown, began to expand in these surroundings.

For the two-year Medical School to grow into a full four-year institution as permitted by legislative action in 1919, a general hospital under the control of the medical faculty was essential. The fulfillment of this paramount need was met by the construction of the Wisconsin General Hospital. However, the location of the hospital left the preclinical branches over in Science Hall remote from patients and the opportunity to correlate more closely their investigations and teaching with the departments of medicine and surgery. To unite the several groups in one center for their major purposes was vitally important.

Again, as had been true for the construction of the Wisconsin General Hospital, surplus funds from the Service Recognition Board were made available by the legislature for the erection of another war memorial. In 1928, the State Laboratory of Hygiene and the several preclinical departments, with the exception of anatomy, moved into the fine laboratories of the Service Memorial Institutes which adjoined the hospital. This building provided space also for the medical library and an adequate auditorium.

A law providing state support for the care of indigent crippled children gave another vital use for the Bradley Hospital. Dr. Bardeen reported that there had been between twenty and twenty-five crippled children in this hospital each day since the law authorizing state support of this work. The crying need for additional hospital facilities to care for these cases appealed strongly to the legislators. Dr. Bardeen worked with unrelenting persistence to secure support and, in 1930, the next structure in the University of Wisconsin Medical Center, the highly attractive Orthopedic Hospital, now Children's Hospital, was completed with state funds. The purpose of the Wisconsin Orthopedic Hospital for Children is defined as follows: "To provide medical, surgical and therapeutic treatment for crippled children under twenty-one years of age whose parents or guardians are unable to provide adequate treatment, or who would be unable otherwise to secure such treatment, these children to remain in said hospital only so long as they can be benefited by this treatment."

Since both the purchasing power of the dollar and personal demands have changed so markedly during the course of this history, I shall give little attention to budgets. The long columns of figures make little sense unless one carries in his mind the rapidly changing curves of values, so any attempt to make accurate comparisons over the decades has, for us, little purpose.

The broad budgetary problems have been considered by Curti and Carstensen with rare appreciation not only of University needs and requests, but also the many demands for every tax dollar and the necessary compromises that each legislative session is forced to make.[2] The periods when the legislators have been relatively favorable to the University have been contrasted with those when other attitudes have prevailed. The period of our special interest, 1904–48, takes us through World War I and II and the serious depression of the 1930's. Manifestly, public neces-

SOURCES OF MONEY AND COST OF BUILDINGS
THE UNIVERSITY OF WISCONSIN MEDICAL SCHOOL THROUGH 1948

BUILDING	YEAR	COST	SOURCE OF FUNDS			
			SPECIAL GRANT	GIFTS	FEDERAL FUNDS	LEGIS-LATURE
BRADLEY MEMORIAL HOSPITAL	1919	93,000		75,000 FROM DR. & MRS. H. C. BRADLEY AND MR. & MRS. C. R. CRANE		18,000
STUDENT INFIRMARY	1919	93,000		50,000 FROM T. E. BRITTINGHAM AND CARL JOHNSON		43,000
ADDITION TO INFIRMARY	1931	98,200	FROM NEW CONSTRUCTION AND SPECIAL FUND (STATE MONEY)			98,200
WISCONSIN GENERAL HOSPITAL	1923	1,110,000	1,110,000 SERVICE RECOGNITION BOARD (STATE MONEY)			
NURSES' DORMITORY	1926	150,200	150,200 SERVICE RECOGNITION BOARD (STATE MONEY)			
SERVICE MEMORIAL INSTITUTES	1928	707,000	707,000 FROM SERVICE RECOGNITION BOARD (STATE MONEY)			
ORTHOPEDIC HOSPITAL	1930	261,000	FROM INSURANCE FUND			261,000
McARDLE LABORATORY	1940	239,993		132,578 FROM McARDLE ESTATE	107,415 (P W A)	

Disbursements for Medical School, Hygienic Laboratory, School of Nursing, and Psychiatric Institute*

	Total Funds	Source of Funds	
		State	Gifts & Trusts
1911–12			
Medical School	$ 37,239.41	$ 37,239.41	
Hygienic Laboratory	8,073.34	8,073.34	
	45,312.75	45,312.75	
1912–13			
Medical School	58,161.95	58,161.95	
Hygienic Laboratory	10,324.08	10,324.08	
	68,486.03	68,486.03	
1919–20			
Medical School	247,193.89	247,193.89	
Hygienic Laboratory	14,481.77	14,481.77	
	261,675.66	261,675.66	
1929–30			
Medical School	348,793.22	342,230.68	$ 6,562.54
School of Nursing	15,931.33	15,931.33	
Psychiatric Institute	37,501.56	37,501.56	
Hygienic Laboratory	37,612.30	37,612.30	
	439,838.41	433,275.87	6,562.54
1939–40			
Medical School	330,227.24	323,688.75	6,538.49
School of Nursing	16,205.87	16,205.87	
Psychiatric Institute	45,772.77	45,772.77	
Hygienic Laboratory	44,006.36	44,006.36	
	436,212.24	429,673.75	6,538.49
1949–50			
Medical School	881,774.84	707,719.83	174,055.01
School of Nursing	34,901.61	34,901.61	
Psychiatric Institute	87,708.34	87,708.34	
Hygienic Laboratory	111,813.21	111,813.21	
	1,116,198.00	942,142.99	174,055.01

*Figures supplied by Neil G. Cafferty, vice-president in charge of business affairs. Large funds from several federal agencies became important after our terminal date.

sities have compelled heavy cuts and vital changes during these periods, and the University took its turn with the rest of the world. On the whole, the citizens of the state have viewed the University with friendly appreciative eyes and have given the needed support.

The small early medical faculty had closer relations with the rest of the University than has been the case during the later periods of increased size and rapid growth. All the members of the early faculty were also members of the College of Letters and Science and served gladly on many University committees.

The legislature, not infrequently, made appropriations to the University on the basis of more than one possible function, leaving, quite properly, the final decision as to the greater need to the authority of the University Board of Regents.

The table on the preceding page shows expenditures for the Medical School in several years during our history. They suggest something of the growth of the school and tremendous changes in the world. To give some idea of the increase in individual salaries, made necessary largely by the diminishing purchasing power of the dollar, the salary of the dean of the Medical School in 1908 was thirty-five hundred dollars; in 1948 it was twelve thousand dollars. In addition, the dean in 1948 had the privilege of consulting and referral practice. In each instance, the dean was professor in an important department; in 1908 he was also chairman of the anatomy department. The salary in each case was for the full year, not the shorter academic year. These figures show roughly a three-fold increase in forty years and are considered more or less representative of the salary changes in the four-decade period.

30 Students and Alumni

We are students of medicine,
    M-E-D-I-C-I-N-E
Where boys schizophrenic and girls neurasthenic
Are happy as galley slaves can be.

We are students of medicine,
    M-E-D-I-C-I-N-E
We dodge staff and nurses, on friends we rehearses
For M-E-D-I-C-I-N-E.

This theme song of our Medichoir, which they rendered with zest and splendid four-part harmony, brings to mind a chorus of the medical students that in less pressing days provided much pleasure both to those who gave and to those who received — a double return that is now missing.

Early in our history, informal warblings — including some close harmonies, premonitions of atonal modern music — were frequently heard in the laboratories; after the Wisconsin General Hospital was completed, festal occasions, such as Christmas, were greeted on the wards by carols sung by nurses, medical students, and residents. Until World War II, *a cappella* group singing increased, initiated by different men as the years rolled around. Dr. Edgar Gordon, coming from a family where music was always a vital part of life both in the home and professionally, brought music into the medical school life in the form of chamber music by a string quartet in which he played the cello and also by choral singing. During World War II, he successfully introduced *a cappella* singing into the 44th Hospital Unit.

In the forties, a splendid quartet consisting of Dick Auerswald, Joseph Freeman, Bob Samp, and Lyle Olson sang for the fun of it. Their spirited singing brought together like-minded students and shortly every Friday at five rehearsals were held under Lyle Olson's able direction, and the Medichoir was born. Competition with similar choral groups, Marquette and others, provided additional incentive, and our Medichoir of over forty voices frequently won first place in these contests. Medigals joined in and a mixed chorus sang for the good fellowship the music provided; few pleasures are more rewarding. Dean Middleton gave the group his blessing. However, times changed (the one thing of which we can be certain), pressures built up, and with the departure of the leader, Lyle Olson, the Medichoir dwindled and, to the regret of all, finally succumbed.

Medical fraternities here at Wisconsin have served another extracurricular function. In the judgment of their faculty advisors and your author, they have commonly contributed to the well-being of their members. The social fraternity attitudes which were appropriate for the academic years have largely been replaced by more serious professional objectives. Much quizzing and teaching of each other within the fraternity has been the mode. Fraternities have given an additional means of contact between faculty and students, much to be desired for both groups. Formerly, most of the medical fraternities supported residential houses; these were lost during the depression of the 1930's; consequently, contacts are now less close. The need of the many married students for fraternity houses and the stimulus of the fraternity is definitely less than for those without these home ties. But despite the social and economic changes, most of the fraternities have kept on and are, to a degree, offsetting somewhat the many centrifugal forces that are confusing both to faculty and to students.

Just as the patient is the most important person in the hospital, so the student occupies a similar position in the medical school. Shortly, he will receive his well-earned doctor of medicine degree, a goal that has seemed so remote and far in the future, and will become an alumnus. In another few years, the alumnus will be practicing the difficult art and the involved science of medicine, either by himself or in some organized clinic.

Back in the autumn of 1914, the University of Wisconsin Medical Society was established with evening meetings held usually in the Science Hall auditorium, for presentation of the results of faculty researches and for guest speakers.[1] Early in the proceedings of this society, a spring meeting was given over to the students for the presentation of some of their investigations.

Incentives for student participation in investigation derive from many sources. In the early days, the support of research was meager; funds from the federal government and foundations were almost nil. All of our students, as members of the College of Letters and Science, were required to present a thesis for the bachelor's degree. Following the Fish curriculum report in 1930, the Letters and Science faculty discontinued the over-all thesis requirement, leaving the decision to the departments. The Medical School continued to require a bachelor's thesis until 1936, and for some years a senior thesis for the M.D. degree was required.

Students who have been part-time assistants in the basic science departments merit special commendation. They immediately became members of the departmental family, taking their share in the duties of teaching, the necessary housework, and the research that was always going on. Partly because the third and fourth years of the medical curriculum were not offered at Wisconsin until 1925, some students took a year off between the second and third years to engage more intensively in research and to earn the master's degree, a splendid rewarding practice that should be continued.

After the Wisconsin General Hospital was completed in 1924 and the Service Memorial Institutes in the summer of 1928, Student Day gradually became a more important function. It was Dr. Bardeen, I think, who suggested holding the student meeting in the daytime. As Student Day grew into an all-day affair, it became a medium of easy fellowship among students and faculty and increasingly a means of presenting the results of the seeding of fertile student minds with the opportunity for research. The papers and the laboratory demonstrations grew better and more varied year by year.

To continue with the lighter side, a noon lunch became part of Student Day, served cafeteria style in one of the laboratories;[2] in the afternoon the students challenged the faculty to a softball game. This was given a boost by Dr. Abe Quisling, who placed a couple of kegs of beer between third base and home plate down in Vilas Park. Both the attendance at the game and the speed of base running increased. It became easier to steal home. Until the senior class became too large, Dr. Quisling generously entertained them all at dinner at the Maple Bluff Country Club, the scene of some of the later ballgames. Of course, the students usually won the game. We seem to have had more football than baseball players among the faculty.

The winning of the game so increased the *amour-propre* of the students that they put on "skits" to take off the foibles of the faculty. This began as a small family affair after a dinner at the Union. It was as easy for a student to portray the professor of obstetrics, Dr. John Harris, with twins or quads and to imitate poorly some of his pungent hyperbole as it was for the one taking the part of skinny Dr. Lew Cole to wrap himself several times in his white coat, cock his head to one side, and dramatically vent his spleen. Of course, the make-believe dean of the period shuffled onto the stage and mumbled some witty response to the proffered red apple, and at a later period, the more military, erect dean tossed back the brown derby exactly onto the head of the offending student. The "skits" grew prodigiously and became an advertised public function in the Union Theater. In a few years the jokes and pantomimes that had at first seemed clever became boring and blatant. The tail wagged the dog so vigorously that the "skits" were discontinued. Possibly they could return as a family affair or have we grown too large and too busy?

Alumni Day also began quite informally. The University Homecoming festivities with gatherings before and after the football games provided the immediate occasions. Alumni dropped in for a chat with their old professors and stayed for exchange of mutual experiences. After the auditorium and laboratories of the Service Memorial Institutes became available in 1928–29, organized programs developed, leading us all along the paths of post-graduate medical education. Excellent programs year after year and the increasing attendance helped to bind faculty, students, and alumni together for common purposes. The programs of the day were commonly followed by a lecture in the evening, at times by a distinguished visitor; frequently, the second day was devoted to clinical demonstrations and discussions.

Of the few printed programs of alumni and student days that have survived to reach the University Archives, that of the meetings held in 1938 with Dr. Harold Bradley as chairman of the committee are rather typical, with Student Day on the 27th and Alumni Day on the 28th of May. As the students are most important, a few items from their program are here included; you will observe that a number of these students have become prominent alumni. Of the twenty-eight student demonstrations shown in laboratories, the following from different departments are representative.

A Demonstration of Bioelectrical Potential with the Cathode Ray Oscillograph — H. L. Bartsch, W. E. Gilson, H. Goldberg.

Gravity Shock — Elizabeth Brodgon, Francis Schaar.

The Effects of Various Sympathicomimetic Drugs on Cardiac Automaticity During Cyclopropane Anesthesia — Jacob W. Stutzman.

The Apparatus for Making Constant Intravenous Injections at Any Desired Rate; Its Use in the Study of the Physiology of Intestinal Smooth Muscle — R. G. Waisman.

An X-Ray Study of the Chest in Various Positions and Phases of Respiration — Bernhard Kaufman, Ben G. Mannis.

X-Ray Studies of the Stomach in Various Positions — L. A. Kregel, Peter B. Golden, Farrell F. Golden, George Grindell, Elmer Steiger.

The Biophotometer — George Hildebrand.

Destruction of Bacteria by Certain Fish Liver Oils — Gordon Worley.

Fish Liver Oil Therapy of Experimental Tuberculosis — Ted Koerner.

Improved Method of Estrogen Assay — H. D. Lauson, C. G. Heiler, J. B. Golden.

The Terrapin Pacemaker in Action — Dr. Frank Maresh.

A Demonstration Illustrating the Mechanism of Urea Clearance — H. J. Nichols.

Organization of the medical alumni was suggested early, but was postponed because the University Alumni Association feared that this would interfere with their long-range projects such as the Union and the Wisconsin Center. However, several of the classes were active in urging an alumni organization, and, as always, a few leaders carried the ball. The class of 1946 published "The Orificial News" as a precursor of our excellent Medical Alumni Association Quarterly. The first and only issue came out in the autumn of 1946 with a youthful picture of Dean Middleton on the front page and a photograph of Ben Lawton as president of the class pressing for a post-intern reunion.

The alumni in the Milwaukee, Rockford, and Madison areas urged strongly the importance of developing an organized alumni association, but this was not accomplished until six to eight years after the terminal date of this history. The account of the bold, far-seeing visions of the University of Wisconsin Medical Alumni Association must therefore be left for the rejoicings of some future historian.[3]

We are such stuff as dreams are made on.
THE TEMPEST

It is to these dreams of the past and to those who have brought them to fruition that this history has been directed. To teaching, to learning, and to service, each member of the faculty has, sometimes with faltering steps, devoted the larger share of his interest and his waking hours. The alumni initiated this history project, this effort to visualize and appreciate our past, its strengths and its difficulties. It is to them, therefore, that I shall address my parting remarks.

With the overwhelming explosions that have been occurring in these recent decades, all persons, whether leaders or followers, have become confused and many patently discouraged. The partial harnessing of nuclear forces, the brilliant flaring of knowledge in many fields, including medicine, the acceptance of the Keynesian economic philosophies by economists and our government, making enormous sums of money available, at least for a period, and most terrifying of all, the stupendous skyrocketing of world population so far beyond available food supplies that both famine and pestilence seem inevitable — all these are requiring vision and new wisdom and new methods, international in scope, to relieve the crushing responsibilities of the leading nations and the dire distress of others.

Surely a species that produces persons who compose and perform glorious moving symphonies and other persons who place Gemini 6 and 7 in orbit and alter their orbits so as to bring the two airships within a few feet of each other while they are moving through the heavens at incredible speed should be able with patience and persistence to avoid the disasters that threaten us.

Chance plays such a vital part in the lives of each one of us that I am choosing some chance words that gave us "the best Commencement speech ever made on this campus." Dean Ingraham, who has enjoyed a good game of tennis for fifty years, missed his footing in a set he was playing at Commencement time in 1948, I think it was. In recovering his balance he slipped and gave his nose a violent whack with the handle of his racket, resulting in widespread red, black, and blue discolorations from the hemorrhage. He disliked the formalities of Commencement so he took advantage of the accident to ask his friend, our distinguished professor of physical chemistry, Farrington Daniels, to act in his stead in presenting the candidates for the bachelor's degree in the College of Letters and Science.

You will all remember the regular procedure and formula from the days when you were receiving your first degree. Professor Daniels, rather excited, instead of inviting the candidates to stand and remain standing, said: "Candidates will please rise and keep rising." After a brief moment the audience burst out with laughter and applause and still more applause as the implications of the remark sank in. As I take my leave of you, I wish to leaven the heavy lump of today's life with this yeast of good will, humor, and tenacity. I charge you *to rise and keep rising.* I have confidence that you will do just that and that you will meet your obligations and your opportunities with courage, a bit of gay laughter, and, I hope, with wisdom.

Reference Material

Notes

1

1 The Jubilee Committee, *The Jubilee of the University of Wisconsin, 1904* (Madison, 1905), p. 223.
2 *Two Lives* (Madison, 1922), p. 1. Bascom Hall originally had a dome similar to that of the Capitol. It was destroyed by fire in 1916.
3 These well-known lines by Sarah N. Cleghorn are quoted here from *Threescore: The Autobiography of Sarah N. Cleghorn* (New York, 1936), p. 161.
4 See Charles McCarthy, *Wisconsin Idea* (New York, 1912).

2

1 Merle Curti and Vernon Carstensen, *The University of Wisconsin, 1848–1925* (Madison, 1949), II, 481.
2 William Snow Miller, Medical schools in Wisconsin: past and present, *Wis. Med. J.* 35:472–86, 1936. William S. Middleton, The first medical faculty of the University of Wisconsin, *Wis. Med. J.* 54:378–85, 1955.
3 *A History of the American Medical Association, 1847–1947* (Philadelphia, 1947), pp. 888–89.
4 *American Medicine* (New York, 1934), p. 123.
5 Middleton, The first medical faculty, p. 379.

3

1 Letter to Charles Bardeen, March 16, 1907.
2 Letter to Senator Burns, Chairman, Joint Committee on Claims, May 17, 1907. The Council on Medical Education of the American Medical Association worked actively for years to improve medical training; but because of states' rights and an aversion to publicity, it was not until after 1908 when they obtained aid from the Carnegie Foundation for the Advancement of Teaching that they were able to achieve notable success. Abraham Flexner and N. P. Colwell of the Council worked intensively for four years and published two startling bulletins, *Medical Education in the United States and Canada* in 1910 and *Medical Education in Europe* in 1912. The results of these reports were astounding, a conspicuous example of the power of well-presented facts to emphasize a great need. These incisive reports, showing the markedly poorer standards of our schools as compared with those in Europe, aroused both state and local

medical associations and generous philanthropists. The development of our own school is part of this broad movement.

3 Joseph Erlanger, A physiologist reminisces, *Ann. Rev. Physiol. 26*:1–14, 1964.
4 In their generous support of the new medical library and in their interest in this history, the two-year graduates have shown their continuing loyalty.
5 Letter to Van Hise, December 15, 1908.
6 Letter to Van Hise, June 17, 1909.
7 Bardeen letter to Van Hise, October 7, 1909.
8 Letter to Dr. John M. Dodson, December 8, 1909.
9 Letter to Regent Edward Evans, January 12, 1910.
10 Letter to Dr. Dodson, December 8, 1909.
11 Undated letter to Dr. Charles Sheldon.
12 See Robert C. Buxbaum and Peter Eichman, A great university and its student health program: an evaluation, *Wis. Med. J. 63*:359–64, 1964. Bardeen letter to Van Hise, January 3, 1910.

4

1 Charles R. Van Hise, The University and the war, *Wis. Alumni Mag.*, November, 1917, pp. 5–7.
2 The only published paper of the experiments was by J. A. E. Eyster and Walter Meek, Experiments on the pathological physiology of acute phosgene poisoning, *Amer. J. Physiol. 51*:303–20, 1920. The study showed that the poisoning produces a well-marked succession of injuries which finally results in typical pulmonary edema. Early injury to the linings of the deep respiratory passages and agglomeration of the red blood cells, which subsequently obstruct the pulmonary capillaries, throwing increased strain on the heart, results in right-sided cardiac dilatation. Death follows from decreased oxygenation of the pulmonary blood.
3 Chauncey D. Leake, letter to author, July, 1964.
4 Major General William L. Sibert, letter to Acting President Birge, December 10, 1918. The sixty-three persons involved in the work are individually mentioned, and sixty-two reports are named by title.
5 February 28, 1919.

5

1 Curti and Carstensen, *The University of Wisconsin*, II, 204.
2 Letter to President Birge, November 24, 1919.
3 *Ibid.*
4 Part of the bill read: "The medical school shall consist of courses of instruction in the medical sciences customarily given in medical schools and may include such additional branches as the Regents may determine." This removed the previous limit to a two-year course and permitted a four-year medical course.

5 *Report upon the Survey of the University of Wisconsin* (Madison, 1915), p. 145.
6 Curti and Carstensen, *The University of Wisconsin*, II, 105.
7 *Ibid.*, 283.
8 Bardeen to W. H. Allen, August 29, 1914.
9 As I look back over the controversies and the attempted or partial blocks in the growth of the Medical School, I find that these many clashes of opinion tend to fade into a hazy picture, just hills and valleys and with sunlight and, at times, deep shadows. Through this half-century and more, the actors and the stage have varied, but the basic reasons for these conflicts have been much the same. Hereafter, in our story, I shall give only the cursory attention to these clashes that they seem to me to merit, as they recede into the past and we learn to live as mature men and women of good will.

6

1 William S. Middleton, The medical preceptorial plan at the University of Wisconsin, *Phi Beta Pi Quarterly* 47:11–16, 1950.
2 For further discussion of the preceptor system, see: C. R. Bardeen, Modern preceptors, *J. Amer. Med. Assoc.* 90:1177–81, 1928; C. R. Bardeen, Extramural clinical teaching: the preceptor system at Wisconsin, *Wis. Med. J.* 27:141–46, 1928; Leslie G. Kindschi, The role of the preceptor in the University of Wisconsin preceptor program, *J. Med. Educ.* 34:649–63, 1959; William S. Middleton, The retirement of preceptors, *Wis. Med. Alumni* 4:10, 1963.
3 Middleton, The medical preceptorial plan, p. 12.
4 John A. Bowers and H. A. Page, Study of a preceptor program, *J. Amer. Med. Assoc.* 173:1923–27, 1960.
5 Unpublished history of the department of medicine by Dr. Ovid Meyer.
6 Lewellys F. Barker, Some tendencies in medical education in the United States, *J. Amer. Med. Assoc.* 57:618–21, 1911.
7 Letter to author, July 13, 1965.

7

1 In October, 1888, after Charles Bardeen had graduated from Syracuse High School, his father took the family to Leipzig, Germany, for a year of study. The father returned to America after the family was well settled. Charles kept a casual diary with brief entries for about seven months. Then he quite wisely states, "There got to be such a sameness in the diary that I left it off on Saturday, the 13th of May." At the beginning of the diary, he stated, "I am a fairly good gymnast, having pulled up to my chin 15 times with all my clothes on. I am a fair scholar, being able to reason better than memorize, and I have a slight mechanical bent." In general, he gives little idea of his inner reactions, although he repeatedly expresses enjoyment of the gymnasium, swimming, fencing, and skating. He also

took mandolin lessons. The European diary of the young Bardeen written in 1888–89 was provided by his son, John Bardeen.

2 Eugene L. Opie, Charles Russell Bardeen, *Bardeen Memorial Laboratories* (Madison, 1957), p. 11.

3 All of these letters were preserved by the family and given to me by William Bardeen with complete permission to use them as seemed appropriate. In general, an enormous amount of material concerning Bardeen is available. I have used conferences with members of his family, letters from his family, many talks with the faculty and former students, my own recollections, as well as Bardeen's printed papers and statements. Manifestly, the final synthesis of all this material is mine, and also the responsibility.

4 Curti and Carstensen, *The University of Wisconsin*, II, 176–79.

5 William Bardeen in personal interview with the author, August 1, 1964.

6 Letter to author, July, 1964.

7 Letter to author, August 12, 1964.

8 Letter to author, October 16, 1964. Dr. TeLinde took his first two years of medicine here, and in 1960 we honored him with the Medical Alumni Citation. For many years he has been distinguished professor of gynecology at Johns Hopkins Medical School.

9 Letter to author, August, 1964.

10 Letter to author, December 10, 1964.

11 Letter to author, July 29, 1964.

12 C. R. Bardeen, On certain visceral pathological alterations, the result of superficial burns, *Bull. Hopkins Hosp.* 8:81–82, 1897. C. R. Bardeen, A review of the pathology of superficial burns with a contribution to our knowledge of the pathological changes in the organs in cases of rapidly fatal burns, *Johns Hopkins Hosp. Rep.* 7:137–79, 1899.

13 C. R. Bardeen, Abnormal development of toad ova fertilized by spermatozoa exposed to the Roentgen rays, *J. Exp. Zool.* 4:1–44, 1907. C. R. Bardeen, Variations in susceptibility of amphibian ova to the X-rays at different stages of development, *Anat. Rec.* 3:638–40, 1909.

14 C. R. Bardeen, Tables for aid in the determination of the relative size of the heart by means of the Roentgen ray, *Amer. J. Roentgen.* 4:604–10, 1917.

<h1 style="text-align:center">8</h1>

1 Curti and Carstensen, *The University of Wisconsin*, II, 490.

2 *Ibid.*

3 He was appointed by the Regents on December 1, 1909, with his duties to begin second semester.

4 William S. Middleton, Memoir of Joseph Spragg Evans, *Trans. Studies Coll. Physicians*, 4th series, *17*:119, 1949.

5 William S. Middleton, conference with the author, August 11, 1964.

6 William Oatway, Altadena, California, letter to author, August, 1964.

7 Jackman Pyre, Tucson, Arizona, letter to author, April 22, 1964.

8 Drs. W. S. Middleton, Karver Puestow, Robin Buerki, and Harry Kay.

9 Letter from Miss Anna Birge, daughter of President Birge, June 4, 1966.

10 Joseph Spragg Evans, Focal infections, *Tice's System of Medicine*. 1920.
J. S. Evans, Epidemiology of acute appendicitis in relation to acute nasal
and tonsillar infections, *Wis. Med. J. 17*:91–93, 1918.
11 Unpublished manuscript in the University of Wisconsin Archives.

9

1 Reminiscenses of Marie Carns, letter to author, July 21, 1964.
2 Dr. Middleton's complete bibliography is available in the University
Archives.
3 William S. Middleton, Palpation of the spleen, *Amer. J. Med. Sci.
167*:118–24, 1924. W. S Middleton and W. H. Oatway, Correlation of
lingual changes with other clinical data, *Arch. Intern. Med. 49*:860–76,
1932. W. S. Middleton, Some clinical caprices of Hodgkin's disease, *Ann.
Intern. Med. 11*:448–68, 1937.
4 This article is typical of Dr. Middleton's strong interest in each patient
and his needs and also of the satisfaction he has derived from his duties
as teacher and clinician. After Dr. Middleton's years (1955–61) as Chief
Medical Director of the Veterans Administration, a highly involved task,
he was appointed acting professor of medicine at the Oklahoma Medical
School with responsibility for patients and teaching on the wards. He
told me, "It was wonderful — like getting back into heaven!"
5 More than any other faculty member, Dr. Middleton has been deeply
interested in the details and progress of this history. He has helped im-
measurably with facts and advice. I have tried rather unsuccessfully to
show him the impossibility of writing such a history with appropriate
contrasting shadows and lights because of personal friendships and social
pressures. Once I said to him, "It would be foolish for me to ask you to
go into the hall and move a ton weight, and it would be unwise for you
to attempt it." Bill looked at me steadfastly a few seconds and then said,
"I'd go out and try." That is, I think, characteristic of Bill Middleton.
Difficult or impossible tasks do not daunt him.

10

1 Arthur J. Patek, A state hygienic laboratory, *Wis. Med. J. 1*:125–26,
1903.
2 Personal conferences with Dr. William D. Stovall, July 13, 1964 and
July 20, 1964.
3 William D. Stovall and M. Starr Nichols, Some factors in swimming pool
control, *J. Infect. Dis. 21*:484–92, 1917.
4 The growth of the laboratory is graphically shown in the increase of
specimens examined, from 2757 in 1906–7 to 174,217 in 1943.
5 W. D. Stovall, Emerald Scheid, and M. Starr Nichols, The influence on
the morphology and staining of *B. diphtheriae* by growth in mixed cultures with staphylococci, and streptococci, *Amer. J. Public Health
13*:748–53, 1923. W. D. Stovall and Mildred Crosswait, Agglutination

reaction in the diagnosis of undulant fever, *Wis. Med. J. 29*:493–97, 1930. W. D. Stovall and Lois Almon, Serological reactions of cultures of Monilia and some other yeast-like fungi, *J. Infect. Dis. 55*:12–25, 1934. Lois Almon, W. D. Stovall, and Jane Read, A study of the Vi anti-genic fraction of typhoid bacilli isolated from carriers and cases, and the antibody content of the serum of these patients, *Amer. J. Public Health 27*:357–62, 1937.

6   Even though it was erected after our terminal date, I must mention the splendid new laboratory building of the State Laboratory of Hygiene, erected through the persistent efforts of Dr. Stovall over several years. Funds were obtained from several sources: the Hill-Burton Fund, the State Board of Health, the University Board of Regents, and, finally, an additional \$300,000 from the Emergency Board. This air-conditioned laboratory is a monument both to Dr. Stovall's persistence and to the deep interest in public health on the part of many governmental agencies.

11

1   Faculty Memorial Committee, Resolutions on the death of Dr. Robert Van Valzah, January 13, 1947, University of Wisconsin Archives, Document 789.

2   Robert Van Valzah, Some deductions from the medical examination of five thousand students entering the University of Wisconsin, *Wis. Med. J. 14*:1–5, 1915. Until the classes became too large, each entering student received a physical examination at the Student Health Service.

3   Robert Van Valzah, Report to the President on influenza epidemic, June 19, 1919. His hypothesis was supported by the work of other physicians: A. G. Love and C. B. Davenport, Immunity of city-bred recruits, *Arch. Intern. Med. 24*:129–53, 1919.

4   Van Valzah, Report to the President, 1919.

5   Edwin O. Jordan, *Epidemic Influenza, a Survey* (Chicago, 1927), p. 214.

6   J. W. Brown, J. L. Sims, E. White, and J. E. Clifford, Liver function during infectious mononucleosis, *Amer. J. Med. 6*:321–28, 1949.

12

1   Baltimore, 1937.

2   Some of us felt these difficulties keenly when Dr. Olaf Larsell, Dr. Miller's younger associate, left us abruptly in 1920. Dr. Larsell's work on the development of the cerebellum is a classic. In addition to tracing its ontogenesis in man, Larsell made a number of comparative studies of the morphogenesis of the cerebellum in other species and related his findings to the physiological data available at the time of his investigations.

3   *Time*, March 15, 1937, p. 60.

4   Frances Hellebrandt, letter to author, February 6, 1965.

5   Clem Nouri, letter to author, February 12, 1965.

6   Walter Sullivan, letter to author, September 29, 1964.
7   Theodore H. Bast and Barry J. Anson, *The Temporal Bone and the Ear* (Springfield, Ill., 1949).
8   George E. Shambaugh, a paper on Theodore H. Bast presented to the Triological Society, January 23, 1965.
9   Frederick D. Geist, Chromatolysis of efferent neurons, *Arch. Neurol. Psychiat. 29*:88–103, 1933.
10 The rabbit placenta and the problem of placental transmission, *Amer. J. Anat. 37*:433–97, 1926.
11 *Contrib. Embryol. 158*:129–246, 1937.
12 Margaret Orsini, letter to author, August, 1964.
13 Mossman, *et al.*, *Human Embryology* (Baltimore, 1945).
14 Otto Mortensen and W. E. Sullivan, The cerebrospinal fluid and the cervical lymph node, *Anat. Rec. 56*:359–63, 1937. Virginia F. Harrison and Otto Mortensen, Identification and voluntary control of single motor unit activity in the tibialis anterior muscle, *Anat. Rec. 144*:109–16, 1962.

13

1   W. J. Meek, *Medico-historical Papers* (Madison, 1954).
2   Letter to author, December 10, 1964. Dr. Haney received his Ph.D. in physiology at Wisconsin in 1934 and his medical degree from the University of Chicago in the same year and is now professor of medicine at the University of Oregon Medical School.
3   Mrs. J. A. E. Eyster, letter to author, July 31, 1964. Other material on Eyster was provided in a letter from Joseph J. and Hensel Lalich, July, 1964, and from Dr. W. S. Middleton's memorial of Dr. Eyster for the Association of American Physicians, July 26, 1960.
4   *Clinical Aspects of Venous Pressure* (New York, 1929). J. A. E. Eyster, The time relations of the venous pulse and the heart sounds, *J. Exp. Med. 14*:594–605, 1911. J. A. E. Eyster and W. J. Meek, The origin and conduction of the heart beat, *Physiol. Rev. 1*:1–43, 1921.
5   Faculty Memorial Resolution, Walter Joseph Meek, April 1, 1963, University of Wisconsin Archives, Document 1582. Faculty Memorial Resolution, John Augustine English Eyster, April 4, 1960, University of Wisconsin Archives, Document 1421.
6   *San Francisco Chronicle*, March 18, 1964.
7   Baltimore, 1935.
8   Ray Herrin and W. J. Meek, Distention as a factor in intestinal obstruction, *Arch. Intern. Med. 51*:152–63, 1933. R. C. Herrin, A. Rabin, R. N. Feinstein, The influence of diet upon urea clearance in the dog, *Amer. J. Physiol. 119*:87–92, 1937. R. C. Herrin and M. Starr Nichols, The influence of vitamin A upon urea and inulin clearance in the dog, *Amer. J. Physiol. 125*:786–801, 1939.
9   F. A. Hellebrandt, Maja Schade, and Marie Carns, Method of evoking the tonic neck reflexes in normal human subjects. *Amer. J. Phys. Med. 41*:90–139, 1962.

10 London, 1949.
11 Eleanor M. Larsen, The fatigue of standing, *Amer. J. Physiol. 150*:109–21, 1947. E. M. Larsen, The menstrual cycle length and variability of young adult women, *Amer. J. Obstet. Gynec. 54*:1069–73, 1947.

14

1 J. H. Kastle and Arthur Loevenhart, The oxidation of formic aldehyde by hydrogen peroxide, *J. Amer. Chem. Soc. 21*:262, 1899. J. H. Kastle and A. S. Loevenhart, Concerning lipase, the fat-splitting enzyme, and the reversibility of its action, *J. Amer. Chem. Soc. 24*:491, 1900.
2 Herbert S. Gasser, Arthur S. Loevenhart, *Science 70*:317–21, 1929.
3 See Harold C. Bradley, Dr. Loevenhart's war work, *Festschrift*: Arthur Loevenhart, 1878–1929, *Phi Beta Pi Quarterly*, November, 1929.
4 A. S. Loevenhart, *Harvey Lectures 10*:85–100, 1915.
5 C. H. Bunting, Personal remembrances of Dr. Loevenhart, *Festschrift*: Arthur Loevenhart, 1878–1929, *Phi Beta Pi Quarterly*, November, 1929.
6 A. L. Tatum and G. A. Cooper, An experimental study of Mapharsen as an antisyphilitic agent, *J. Pharmacol. Exp. Ther. 50*:198–215, 1934.
7 Frederick E. Shideman, A. L. Tatum, practical pharmacologist, *Science 123*:449, 1956.
8 B. J. Longley, N. M. Clausen, and A. L. Tatum, Cultivation of various species of trypanosomes in the developing chick embryo, *Proc. Soc. Exp. Biol. Med. 41*:365–66, 1939.
9 M. H. Seevers, letter to author, January 29, 1965.
10 Shideman, A. L. Tatum, p. 449.
11 *The Old Egyptian Medical Papyri* (Lawrence, Kansas, 1952). *Yellow Fever in Galveston, Republic of Texas, 1839* (Austin, Texas, 1951).

15

1 C. H. Bunting and John Lawrence Yates, Cultural results in Hodgkin's disease, *Arch. Intern. Med. 12*:236–42, 1913. C. H. Bunting, Hodgkin's disease, *Bull. Hopkins Hosp. 25*:173–80, 1914.
2 Gorton Ritchie, letter to author, July 18, 1964.
3 Otto Mortensen, letter to author, January, 1965.
4 C. H. Bunting, letter to author, 1960.
5 C. H. Bunting and John Huston, The fate of the lymphocyte, *J. Exp. Med. 33*:593–600, 1921. C. H. Bunting and Henry Bunting, Acid mucopolysaccharides of the aorta, *Arch. Path. 55*:257–64, 1953.
6 E. M. Medlar, *The Behavior of Pulmonary Tuberculosis Lesions* (New York, 1955).
7 *Arch. Path. 38*:123–27, 1944.
8 *Wis. Med. J. 35*:790–98, 1938.
9 John McCarter, letter to author, January 17, 1965.
10 *Amer. J. Med. Sci. 196*:796–814, 1958.

11 D. Murray Angevine, R. L. Cecil, Sidney Rothbard, Influence of various types of immunization on the genesis of experimental hemolytic streptococcus arthritis, *Arch. Path.* *34*:18–30, 1942.

16

1 A physiologist reminisces, *Ann. Rev. Physiol.* *26*:7–8, 1964.
2 Harold C. Bradley, Reminiscences of Doctor Bardeen, *Bardeen Memorial Laboratories*, pp. 17–22.
3 *Ibid.*
4 Letter to author, April 27, 1964.
5 Curti and Carstensen, *The University of Wisconsin*, II, 485.
6 Russell H. Chittenden, *The Development of Physiological Chemistry in the United States* (New York, 1930), pp. 206–11.
7 H. C. Bradley, Autolysis and atrophy, *Physiol. Rev.* *2*:415–39, 1922.
8 H. C. Bradley and David R. Brower, Roads in the national parks, *Sierra Club Bulletin*, June, 1960.
9 *Enzymologia 2*:265–84, 1942.
10 Philip P. Cohen and M. Hyano, Urea synthesis by liver homogenates, *J. Biol. Chem.* *166*:239–50, 1946.
11 H. F. Deutsch, R. A. Alberty, and L. J. Gosting, Separation and purification of a new globulin from normal human plasma, *J. Biol. Chem.* *165*:21–35, 1946.

17

1 A fine letter from Dr. John Parks, chiefly about John Harris, suggests that someone should write a biographical sketch of the author. Others have made the same suggestion; but during the ordeal of this history, I have found that composing a biography of a friend still living is so difficult that I could not bring myself to make such a request of anyone. The story of Paul F. Clark is, therefore, autobiographical; I am indeed sorry. With humility, I was indeed happy to receive the citation given to me by the Medical Alumni Association in 1961. It was a deciding factor in inducing me to undertake this history.
2 *Alice in Virusland* (Madison, 1938), originally published in *J. Bact.* *36*:223–41, 1938. Paul F. Clark and Alice S. Clark, *Memorable Days in Medicine* (Madison, 1942). Paul F. Clark, *Pioneer Microbiologists of America* (Madison, 1961).
3 *Aphorisms* (New York, 1950), p. 36.
4 D. F. Pettibone, E. B. Bogart, and P. F. Clark, The bacteriology of the bubble fountain, *J. Bact.* *1*:471–80, 1916.
5 Paul F. Clark and Alice S. Clark, A bacteriophage active against a virulent hemolytic streptococcus, *Proc. Soc. Exp. Biol. Med.* *24*:635–39, 1927.
6 Catalog of the University of Wisconsin, 1920–21, p. 353.

7   Curti and Carstensen, *The University of Wisconsin*, II, 488.

8   The placental transmission of foreign proteins in rabbits, *J. Immun.* *19*:177–216, 1930. Antibody response to hemoglobin absorbed on aluminum hydroxide, *J. Immun.* *46*:47–58, 1943.

9   Hobart W. Cromwell, Quantitative relations in the precipitin reaction, *J. Infect. Dis.* *37*:321–28, 1925.

10   Capsules in young cultures of Streptococcus hemolyticus, *J. Bact.* *28*:481–87, 1934. Hemolytic streptococcus lymphadenitis in guinea pigs, *J. Exp. Med.* *70*:347–59, 1939.

11   A. F. Rasmussen, Jr., H. A. Waisman, C. A. Elvehjem, and P. F. Clark, Influence of the level of thiamine intake on the susceptibility of mice to poliomyelitis virus, *J. Infect. Dis.* *74*:41–47, 1944.

18

1   He perfected one of the early quantitative Wassermann tests and later a flocculation reaction for syphilis that proved highly accurate. He delighted in this type of work.

2   Letter from Lorenz to Bardeen, February 10, 1916.

3   A. S. Loevenhart, W. F. Lorenz, H. G. Martin, and J. Y. Malone, Stimulation of the respiration by sodium cyanide and its clinical application, *Arch. Intern. Med.* *21*:109–29, 1918.

4   A. S. Loevenhart, W. F. Lorenz, and R. M. Waters, Cerebral stimulation, *J. Amer. Med. Assoc.* *92*:880–83, 1929.

5   Letter to author from Dr. Mabel G. Masten, June 9, 1965.

6   Fifth biennial report of the Wisconsin Psychiatric Institute, 1924.

7   University of Wisconsin Catalog, 1948–50, pp. 506–7.

8   All three men were athletes in college. Reese played soccer in the Olympic Games of 1912. All three served their countries in World War I. Lorenz had served in the Spanish-American War also and tried unsuccessfully to enter the armed forces in World War II. Bleckwenn was in World War I in the ROTC and served with distinction as Commanding Officer of the 135th Medical Regiment in World War II. Reese served with U.S. forces during World War II as a combat scientist (1943–45) in England and France.

9   Hans Reese, Nonspecific and malarial therapy in neurosyphilis, *Amer. J. Syph.* *13*:348–59, 1929.

10   W. F. Lorenz, A. S. Loevenhart, W. J. Bleckwenn, and F. J. Hodges, The therapeutic use of tryparsamide in neurosyphilis, *J. Amer. Med. Assoc.* *81*:1497–1502, 1923.

11   W. J. Bleckwenn, Sodium amytal in certain nervous and mental conditions, *Wis. Med. J.* *29*:693–96, 1930.

12   W. C. Menninger, *Psychiatry in a Troubled World* (New York, 1948), p. 310.

13   Two of the greatest American leaders in public hygiene, Dr. Hermann M. Biggs and Dr. William Park, were both on the Bellevue faculty while Lorenz was a student there. With my knowledge of these two men, I can

hardly imagine that they failed to pass on some of their public health zeal to the young Lorenz.

14 William F. Lorenz, Clinical notes on pellagrins receiving an excessive diet, *Public Health Rep.* 29:2357–63, 1914.

15 W. J. Bleckwenn and Mabel G. Masten, Antidotal treatment of barbiturate intoxication, *J. Amer. Med. Assoc.* 111:504–7, 1938.

16 Letter from William J. Bleckwenn to Hans H. Reese, August 25, 1964. Dr. Reese has also provided me with an unpublished biography of Dr. Bleckwenn.

17 Mabel G. Masten and R. C. Bunts, Neurogenic erosions and perforations of the stomach and esophagus in cerebral lesions, *Arch. Intern. Med.* 54:916–30, 1934.

18 Annette C. Washburne, Bromism, *Wis. Med. J.* 33:746–50, 1934.

19 Fritz Kant, *The Treatment of the Alcoholic* (Springfield, 1952).

19

1 Ovid Otto Meyer, G. E. Stewart, E. W. Thewlis, and H. P. Rusch, The hypophysis and hematopoiesis, *Folia Haemat.* 57:99–109, 1937. J. B. Bingham, O. O. Meyer, and F. J. Pohle, Studies on the hemorrhagic agent 3, 3-methylenebis (4-hydroxycoumarin), *Amer. J. Med. Sci.* 202:563–78, 1941. O. O. Meyer, Historical data regarding the experiences with coumarin anticoagulants at the University of Wisconsin Medical School, *Circulation* 19:114–17, 1959.

2 E. W. Thewlis and O. O. Meyer, The blood count of normal white rats, *Anat. Rec.* 82:115–25, 1942.

3 Letter to author, August 3, 1965.

4 *Symposium on the Blood and Blood-forming Organs* (Madison, 1939).

5 Dr. Meyer's eighteen-page unpublished manuscript on the history of the department of medicine has been most helpful and gives details that my broader history has been compelled to omit. Would that each department had followed Dr. Meyer's splendid example!

6 *Orthodiascopy* (New York, 1937).

7 The department of physiology records the early purchase of a large string galvanometer from Edelman that arrived September 24, 1911. It cost $6050.98; where did such an incredible amount of money come from? Professor Einthoven visited Dr. Eyster in 1924.

8 Herman H. Shapiro and Leo A. Smyth, Transient electrocardiographic changes noted during attacks of angina pectoris with report of a case, *J. Lab. Clin. Med.* 23:819–22, 1938. Herman H. Shapiro, Treatment of congestive heart-failure, *Wis. Med. J.* 20:237–40, 1956.

9 Karl Paul Link, The anticoagulant from spoiled sweet clover hay, *Harvey Lectures* 34:162–216, 1943–44. Ovid O. Meyer, Historical data regarding the experiences with coumarin anticoagulants at the University of Wisconsin Medical School, *Circulation* 19:114–17, 1959.

10 A. L. Tatum and G. A. Cooper, Mapharsen as an antisyphilitic agent, *Science* 75:541–42, 1932. A. L. Tatum and G. A. Cooper, An experi-

mental study of Mapharsen as an antisyphilitic agent, *J. Pharmacol. Exp. Ther. 50*:198–215, 1934.

11 O. H. Foerster, R. L. McIntosh, L. M. Wieder, H. R. Foerster, and G. A. Cooper, Mapharsen in the treatment of syphilis, *Arch. Dermatol. Syphilol. 32*:868–92, 1935. L. M. Wieder, O. H. Foerster, and H. R. Foerster, Mapharsen in the treatment of syphilis, further experiences, *Arch. Dermatol. Syphilol. 35*:402–13, 1937.

12 P. A. Duehr, L. L. Weismiller, R. L. McIntosh, G. A. Cooper, and A. L. Tatum, Mapharsen, a new therapeutic agent for Vincent's infection, *J. Amer. Dent. Assoc. 23*:652–53, 1936.

13 Memorial resolutions of the faculty on the death of Dr. Roscoe Lyle McIntosh, February 2, 1953, University of Wisconsin Archives, Document 1071.

14 U. J. Wile and Sture A. M. Johnson, Use of splenectomized and non-splenectomized mice in the production of experimental syphilis in rabbits, *Amer. J. Syphil. 28*:422–30, 1944. S. A. M. Johnson and A. R. Test, Epidermolysis bullosa simplex of the hands and feet, *Arch. Dermatol. Syphilol. 53*:610–19, 1946.

15 Ray C. Blankinship, Peptic ulcer, *Wis. Med. J. 28*:294–98, 1929: Modern methods of diagnosis in gastrointestinal disorders, *Wis. Med. J. 28*:593–97, 1929.

16 Karver L. Puestow, The role of bacteria in the gastrointestinal tract with changing concepts of intestinal function, *Amer. J. Gastroent. 25*:22–32, 1956.

17 K. L. Puestow, Maduromycosis, *Arch. Dermatol. Syphilol. 20*:642–64, 1929.

18 Elmer L. Sevringhaus, letter to author, November 5, 1964.

19 E. L. Sevringhaus, The minimum ascorbic acid needs of adults, *J. Nutr. 27*:271–85, 1944.

20 E. L. Sevringhaus, *Endocrine Therapy in General Practice* (Chicago, 1945).

21 Memorial resolutions of the faculty on the death of Dr. John E. Gonce, Jr., May 7, 1956, University of Wisconsin Archives, Document 1223.

22 John E. Gonce, Jr., and Karl Kassowitz, Effect of ultraviolet light on the bacteriological property of whole blood, *J. Amer. Med. Assoc. 20*:280–84, 1928. J. E. Gonce and H. L. Templeton, Citric acid milk in infant feeding, *Amer. J. Dis. Child. 39*:265–76, 1939.

23 H. Kent Tenney, Jr., *Let's Talk About Your Baby* (Minneapolis, 1934).

24 H. K. Tenney, Jr., The prevention of behavior problems in children, *J. Pediat. 19*:833–40, 1941.

25 Kenneth B. McDonough, The treatment of meningitis, *Wis. Med. J. 46*:703–7, 1947. K. B. McDonough and D. R. Borgen, A study of the relation of rickets to anemia, *J. Lab. Clin. Med. 22*:819–24, 1937.

26 Harry Waisman, Production of riboflavin deficiency in the monkey (Macaca mulatta), *Proc. Soc. Exp. Biol. Med. 55*:69–71, 1944. Waisman, *et al.*, Studies on the nutritional requirements of the Rhesus monkey, *J. Nutr. 26*:205–18, 1943.

27 R. H. Stiehm, Tuberculous infections and progressive tuberculous lesions, *Lancet 57*:33–34, 1937.

28 J. McCarter, H. R. Getz, and R. H. Stiehm, A comparison of intra-

cutaneous reactions in man to the purified protein derivatives of several species of acid fast bacteria, *Amer. J. Med. Sci. 195*:479–93, 1938.

29 H. M. Coon, The 7th floor, *Crusader 51*:7–9, 1958. This seventh-floor ward was both well isolated and attractive. The murals "dreamed up" by Dr. Oatway, studied in detail and painted by his sister Margarette (Mrs. C. H. Dornbusch), presented colorfully the diagnosis and treatment of tuberculosis through the ages.

30 Dr. Oatway was both a patient and a research fellow at Saranac. He used his time not only to get well but also to carry on investigations with Drs. Steenken and Petroff. William H. Oatway, Jr., Correlation of leucocyte interpretation of Medlar with the clinical findings of pulmonary tuberculosis, *Amer. Rev. Tuberc. 21*:786–810, 1930; W. H. Oatway, Jr., S. A. Petroff, and W. Steenken, Jr., Biological studies of tubercle bacillus, *J. Exp. Med. 60*:515–40, 1934.

31 W. H. Oatway, Jr., Progress of the University of Wisconsin Medical School — The years before 1923, unpublished manuscript, University of Wisconsin Medical Library.

32 Helen A. Dickie, Spontaneous mediastinal emphysema and spontaneous pneumothorax, a report of 20 cases, *Ann. Intern. Med. 28*:618–29, 1948.

33 Marie L. Carns and Annette C. Washburne, Psychiatric investigation in internal medicine, *Ann. Intern. Med. 7*:664–68, 1933.

34 Frederick J. Pohle, The blood platelet count in relation to the menstrual cycle in normal women, *Amer. J. Med. Sci. 197*:40–47, 1939. F. J. Pohle and John J. Stewart, The cephalin cholesterol flocculation reaction as an aid in the diagnosis of hepatic disorders, *J. Clin. Invest. 20*:241–47, 1941.

35 J. L. Sims, Multiple bilateral pulmonary adenomatosis in man, *Arch. Intern. Med. 71*:403–9, 1943.

20

1 Many sets of journals, such as *Zeitschrift für Hygiene, Annales de l'Institut Pasteur,* and *Centralblat für Bakteriologie,* were present in the several University libraries.

2 Dr. Bardeen spent the larger part of a year working over the detailed plans for the Service Memorial Institutes. He handled details of equipment usually delegated to architects and their aides.

3 From these painstaking displays grew the book, *Memorable Days in Medicine* (Madison, 1942), which she co-authored with Dr. Clark. For some years Mrs. Clark also instructed first-year medical students in small groups in the use of the library and its bibliographical aids. All this was volunteer work.

4 William S. Middleton, The Medical Library of the University of Wisconsin, a talk presented May 6, 1958, to the Wisconsin Medical Alumni Association. He lists many gifts which we cannot take space to acknowledge.

5 In setting a value on this library, J. Christian Bay, librarian of the John Crerar Library, Chicago, commented in his inventory of the collection, "Owing to his ingenuity as a bibliophile of medical literature, Professor

Miller, during his long life, was able to accumulate a library quite unusually complete, important, and comprehensive."

6 Helen Crawford, Regional plans for medical library service, *Bull. Med.
Libr. Assoc. 53*:514–19, 1964.

21

1 Frederick J. Gaenslen, Sacroilia arthrodesia, *J. Amer. Med. Assoc.
89*:2031–35, 1927. F. J. Gaenslen, Congenital defects of the tibia and
fibula, *Amer. J. Orth. Surg. 12*:453–79, 1914. F. J. Gaenslen, Osteitis
deformans (Paget's disease), *Amer. J. Orth. Surg. 13*:96–117, 1915.

2 Robert E. Burns, An osteoperiosteal chisel, *J. Bone Joint Surg. 23*:384–
85, 1941. R. E. Burns, Osteomyelitis: a study of 162 cases treated by
the Orr method, *Wis. Med. J. 30*:982–84, 1931.

3 George Van Ingen Brown, *The Surgery of Oral Diseases and Malformations* (New York, 1912). G. V. I. Brown, The surgical treatment of post-
operative lip and palate defects, *J. Amer. Med. Assoc. 62*:1539–41, 1914.
G. V. I. Brown, Readjustment of the superior maxillae in the treatment
of harelip and cleft palate, *J. Amer. Med. Assoc. 52*:1026–31, 1909.

4 An undated letter from Dr. Brown to Dr. Hyslop gives some of the personal story: "Notwithstanding the fact that it was necessary to be up at
four and on the road at five o'clock in the morning in order to get breakfast and be in the hospital by eight o'clock, I nevertheless became deeply
interested in the University work. I enjoyed the contacts with medical
students and nurses that my lectures gave me, my clinics before students,
and the operating appointments that the University offered as the number
of patients continued to increase. . . ."

5 Volney B. Hyslop, A cleft palate repair technique affording better speech
results, *Wis. Med. J. 36*:540–43, 1937.

6 In the case of Dr. Hedblom, I have ignored my seven-year residence rule
because he was our first and highly competent full-time professor of
surgery and because his service here shows that many factors aside from
immediate professional competence are essential, especially in a young
institution not yet well established.

7 Erwin R. Schmidt, Forty-four cases of simple perforation of gastric and
duodenal ulcers with a simple method of surgical treatment, *Acta Chir.
Scand. 55*:313–42, 1923. E. R. Schmidt, Burns, *Amer. J. Surg. 8*:274–76,
1930.

8 Unpublished papers on Paracelsus read at the Miller medical history
seminars in 1928, 1929, and 1930.

9 Kenneth Elroy Lemmer and J. P. Malec, Drainage of the common bile
duct with resultant extrarenal azotemia, *Arch. Surg. 39*:125–30, 1939.
K. E. Lemmer, Carcinoid tumors of the stomach, *Surgery 12*:378–82,
1942.

10 Anthony R. Curreri and Joseph W. Gale, Decortication in the treatment
of chronic empyema, *Arch. Surg. 55*:486–92, 1947, A. R. Curreri and
J. W. Gale, Mediastinal tumors, *Arch. Surg. 58*:797–817, 1949.

11 Joseph W. Gale, F. A. Hidde, and J. P. Malec, Carcinoma of the breast,
Amer. J. Surg. 49:427–33, 1940. J. W. Gale, A. R. Curreri, and B. J.

Longley, Experiences with pulmonary resection, paper given at the 53rd Annual Meeting of the Western Surgical Association, Chicago, 1945. J. W. Gale, The present status of pulmonary resection in the treatment of pulmonary tuberculosis, *Surg. Gynec. Obstet.* 87:751–53, 1948.

12 Ira R. Sisk, J. B. Wear, and H. A. O'Brien, Transplantation of the ureters to the sigmoid, *Surg. Gynec. Obstet.* 52:212–22, 1931. I. R. Sisk and J. B. Wear, Gonococcal infections of the kidneys, ureter and bladder, *J. Urol.* 23:639–59, 1930. I. R. Sisk and J. B. Wear, Gonococcal pyelonephritis, *Urol. Cutan. Rev.* 40:390–93, 1936.

13 Conferences with Dr. John B. Wear, Jr.

14 Frederick Allison Davis, What the general practitioner should know about ophthalmoscopic examinations, *Postgrad. Med.* 4:473–500, 1948. Primary tumors of the optic nerve, *Arch. Ophthal.* 23:735–41, 1940.

15 Peter A. Duehr, Some primary considerations in retinal detachment, *Wis. Med. J.* 46:515–19, 1947.

16 Wellwood M. Nesbit, L. W. Paul, and W. S. Middleton, Congenital aplasia of the lung. *Amer. J. Roentgen.* 57:446–48, 1947.

17 Wilder Penfield and Theodore C. Erickson, *Epilepsy and Cerebral Localization* (Springfield, 1941). T. C. Erickson, What types of epileptiform-like seizures are amenable to surgical treatment, *Amer. J. Dis. Child.* 75:712–20, 1948. G. W. Newall, T. C. Erickson, W. E. Gilson, S. N. Geishoff, and C. A. Elvehjem, Studies on human subjects receiving highly agenized food materials, *J. Lab. Clin. Med.* 34:239–45, 1949.

18 F. E. Mohs and M. F. Guyer, Pre-excisional fixation of tissues in the treatment of cancer in rats, *Cancer Res.* 1:49–51, 1941. F. E. Mohs, Chemosurgery: a microscopically controlled method of cancer excision, *Arch. Surg.* 42:279–95, 1941.

19 F. E. Mohs, Chemosurgical treatment of the skin: a microscopically controlled method of excision, *J. Amer. Med. Assoc.* 138:546–69, 1948. F. E. Mohs, *Chemosurgery in Cancer, Gangrene and Infections* (Springfield, 1956).

22

1 Carl S. Harper, A self-retaining cannula for injection of liquids or gas in tubal insufflation, *Amer. J. Obstet. Gynec.* 16:892–93, 1926. C. S. Harper and O. N. Anderson, Congenital defects of the diaphragm with relation to asphyxia neonatorum, *Amer. J. Obstet. Gynec.* 20:324–51, 1930.

2 Harry Rosenfeld and Edwin F. Schneiders, Improved phenoltetrachlorphthalein test in the toxemias of pregnancy, *J. Amer. Med. Assoc.* 80:743–47, 1923. E. F. Schneiders, More than 5,500 consecutive maternity cases without a maternal death from any cause, *Amer. J. Obstet. Gynec.* 58:342, 1949.

3 Letter to author from Curtis J. Lund, February 2, 1965.

4 John W. Harris and J. H. Brown, A clinical and bacteriological study of 113 cases of streptococcic puerperal infection, *Bull. Hopkins Hosp.* 44:1–31, 1929. J. W. Harris, Three cases of streptococcic puerperal infection with unusual lesions, *Bull. Hopkins Hosp.* 43:26–32, 1928.

5   Ralph M. Waters and J. W. Harris, Carbon dioxide and oxygen problems in obstetric anesthesia, *Anesth. Analg. 10*:56–63, 1931.

6   Ralph E. Campbell, Treatment of pelvic tuberculosis in the female by radiation therapy, based upon experimental evidence in the animal and clinical results in the human (a five-year study), *Trans. Amer. Assoc. Obstet. Gynec. Abdom. Surg. 57*:56–73, 1946. R. E. Campbell and E. L. Sevringhaus, Pituitary gonadotropic extract for treatment of amenorrhea, menorrhagia, and sterility, *Amer. J. Obstet. Gynec. 37*:913–28, 1939.

7   Madeline J. Thornton, The use of vaginal tampons for the absorption of menstrual discharge, *Amer. J. Obstet. Gynec. 46*:259–65, 1947.

23

1   Fred J. Hodges and J. A. E. Eyster, Estimation of transverse cardiac diameter in man, *Arch. Intern. Med. 37*:704–14, 1926.

2   E. A. Pohle, Studies of the roentgen erythema of the human skin, *Radiology 6*:236–45, 1926. E. A. Pohle and E. L. Sevringhaus, Studies of the systematic effect of roentgen rays, *Amer. J. Roentgen. 23*:291–98, 1930.

3   E. A. Pohle, *Clinical Roentgen Therapy* (Philadelphia, 1938). E. A. Pohle, *Theoretical Principles of Roentgen Therapy* (Philadelphia, 1938). E. A. Pohle, *Clinical Radiation Therapy* (Philadelphia, 1950).

4   Lester W. Paul, Roentgen diagnosis of carcinoma of the pancreas, *Amer. J. Cancer 28*:34–72, 1936. L. W. Paul and E. A. Pohle, Solitary myeloma of bone, *Radiology 36*:651–66, 1940. L. W. Paul and G. Ritchie, Pulmonary adenomatosis, *Radiology 47*:334–43, 1946. L. W. Paul and J. H. Juhl, Pulmonary adenomatosis: further roentgen observations, *Radiology 55*:681–91, 1950. L. W. Paul and J. H. Juhl, *The Essentials of Roentgen Interpretation* (New York, 1959).

24

1   Ralph M. Waters, Pioneering in anesthesiology, *Postgrad. Med. 4*:265–70, 1948.

2   Anesthesiology was officially a part of the department of surgery until after Dr. Waters retired. It was, however, a working unit, and it seems appropriate to place Dr. Waters, his associates, and their contributions in a separate chapter. The term "department" has been used loosely by many persons, including Dean Bardeen, both in oral and written reports. I have followed his example. "Subdepartment" and "division" are also terms that have been used with different connotations at different periods in our history.

3   Letter to author, April, 1965. I received several delightful letters from Dr. Waters in March and April, 1965.

4   Waters, Pioneering in anesthesiology, p. 267.

5   Noel A. Gillespie, Ralph Milton Waters: a brief biography, *Brit. J. Anaesth. 21*:201–2, 1949.

6   R. M. Waters, Present status of cyclopropane, *Brit. Med. J.* 2:1013–17, 1936.

7   R. M. Waters, R. H. Fitch, and A. L. Tatum, The intravenous use of the barbituric acid hypnotics in surgery, *Amer. J. Surg.* 9:110–14, 1930. R. M. Waters and C. Leake, Anesthetic properties of carbon dioxide, *Anesth. Analg.* 8:17–19, 1929.

8   N. A. Gillespie, *Endotracheal Anaesthesia* (Madison, 1950).

9   Ralph M. Waters, ed., *Chloroform: A Study After 100 Years* (Madison, 1951).

10 Gillespie, Ralph Milton Waters: a brief biography, p. 202.

11 Resolutions of the faculty, November 7, 1955, University of Wisconsin Archives, Document 1189.

12 R. M. Waters, O. S. Orth, and N. A. Gillespie, Trichlorethylene anesthesia and cardiac rhythm, *Anesthesiology* 4:1–5, 1943. O. S. Orth, M. D. Leigh, C. H. Mellish and J. W. Stutzman, Action of sympathomimetic amines in cyclopropane, ether and chloroform anesthesia, *J. Pharmacol. Exp. Ther.* 67:1–16, 1939.

13 Resolutions of the faculty, May 4, 1964, University of Wisconsin Archives, Document 1625.

25

1   Articles by Bardeen on the hospital include: State of Wisconsin General Hospital opens at Madison; general policies are outlined, *Wis. Med. J.* 23:211–16, 1924; The teaching hospital and the medical school, *Proc. Cong. Med. Educ.* (Chicago, 1929).

2   *Wisconsin Statutes Relating to the University Hospitals* (Madison, 1954).

3   Conference with Mrs. Walter Schulte (Helen Denne), April 9, 1965.

4   *Graduate Medical Education* (Chicago, 1940).

5   Harry D. Bouman, Electrical stimulation of respiration, *Amer. J. Phys. Med.* 31:40–52, 1952. H. D. Bouman, D. I. Briggs, and A. E. Harris, The value of relaxation procedures in the treatment of anxiety tension states, *Occup. Ther. Rehab.* 29:345–53, 1950.

6   William Osler, *Aequanimitas* (Philadelphia, 1947), p. 255.

26

1   *Nursing and Nursing Education in the United States* (New York, 1923).

2   Conference with Mrs. Walter Schulte (Helen Denne), April 9, 1965.

3   *Obstetrical Nursing* (New York, 1957).

27

1   H. P. Rusch, Cancer research at the University of Wisconsin, an unpublished manuscript (written in 1942) in the University of Wisconsin Archives. The later development of cancer research at the University is

detailed in Charles A. Culotta's The growth of the McArdle Laboratory for Cancer Research, an unpublished manuscript written in 1965.

2   H. P. Rusch, B. E. Kline, and C. A. Baumann, Carcinogenesis by ultra-violet rays with reference to wave length and energy, *Arch. Path.* *31*:135–46, 1941.

3   H. P. Rusch, B. E. Kline, and C. A. Baumann, The influence of caloric restriction and of dietary fat on tumor formation with ultra-violet radiation, *Cancer Res. 5*:431–35, 1945.

4   D. L. Miner, J. A. Miller, C. A. Baumann, and H. P. Rusch, The effect of pyridoxin and other B-vitamins on the production of liver cancer with p-dimethylaminoazobenzene, *Cancer Res. 3*:296–302, 1943. E. C. Miller, C. A. Baumann, and H. P. Rusch, Certain effects of dietary pyridoxine and casein on the carcinogenicity of p-dimethylaminoazobenzene, *Cancer Res. 5*:713–16, 1945.

5   Van R. Potter, The assay of animal tissues for respiratory enzymes, *J. Biol. Chem. 169*:17–37, 1947.

6   K. P. DuBois and V. R. Potter, Biocatalysts in cancer tissues, *Cancer Res. 2*:290–93, 1942.

7   E. C. Miller and J. A. Miller, The presence and significance of bound aminoazo dyes on the livers of rats fed para-dimethylaminoazobenzene, *Cancer Res. 7*:468–80, 1947.

28

1   University of Wisconsin news release, March, 1949.
2   *War Without Guns*, pp. 16, 20, 25.
3   From conversations with many faculty members, especially Dean Mark Ingraham and Dr. Anthony Curreri, it seems clear that we owe a vast debt to President E. B. Fred for his persuasive skill in emphasizing that this Memorial Library would be a wonderful, growing memorial of great service to the University and the future citizens of the state. Unfortunately, shortages of metal because of the war made it impossible to construct the spandrils of bronze which would have picked up the color of the massive pink granite entrance and carried this color to the top of the building.

29

1   Bardeen to Van Hise, June 28, 1917.
2   Aside from remarks here and there throughout the two volumes, special attention is given to money matters in three chapters under the titles of "Getting and Spending." In Volume I, Chapter 21 presents the problems of 1887–1903; in Volume II, Chapter 5 considers those of 1903–14 and Chapter 6 the period from 1914–25.

30

1 The first meetings of the University of Wisconsin Medical Society were held in Room 210 of the Chemical Engineering Building; later, from about 1917–27, meetings were held in the auditorium of Science Hall. Since 1928, the formal meetings of the society, as well as those on Alumni Day and Student Day, have taken place in the auditorium of Service Memorial Institutes. World War II put an end to the regular meetings of the University of Wisconsin Medical Society. After the war, public general medical staff meetings have been held about once a month, usually in the SMI auditorium at noon. Frequently, visiting lecturers have presented their contributions at this hour.

2 The first lunch — plenty of good baked ham — was prepared by two of our students, Myra Emery (Burke) and Emma Brindley (Kyhos). Later, the lunches were prepared by the hospital staff.

3 The Alumni Association's most dramatic achievement has been the new medical library. The funds were obtained from the following sources: Alumni, faculty, and friends, $700,000; State of Wisconsin, $300,000; Brittingham Estate, $200,000; Lewis E. Phillips, Eau Claire, $50,000. These estimates were provided in a letter from Neil Cafferty, January 20, 1967.

Index